THE Beans
Lentils
&Tofu
GOURMET

THE Beans Lentils & Tofu GOURMET

The Beans, Lentils and Tofu Gourmet

For complete cataloguing information, see page 6.

DESIGN, EDITORIAL AND PRODUCTION:	MATTHEWS COMMUNICATIONS DESIGN INC.
PHOTOGRAPHY:	MARK T. SHAPIRO
ART DIRECTION, FOOD PHOTOGRAPHY:	SHARON MATTHEWS
FOOD STYLIST:	KATE BUSH
PROP STYLIST:	CHARLENE ERRICSON
MANAGING EDITOR:	PETER MATTHEWS
INDEX:	BARBARA SCHON
COLOR SCANS & FILM:	POINTONE GRAPHICS

Cover image: Gamberi e fagioli alla Massimo *(Massimo's shrimp and beans), Page 121*

We acknowledge the financial support of the Government of Canada through the Book Publishing Industry Development Program (BPIDP) for our publishing activities.
Canadä

Published by: Robert Rose Inc. • 120 Eglinton Ave. E., Suite 1000
Toronto, Ontario, Canada M4P 1E2 Tel: (416) 322-6552

Printed in Canada
1234567 BP 03 02 01 00

Contents

Canadian Cataloguing in Publication Data

The beans, lentils and tofu gourmet

Includes index.
ISBN 0-7788-0023-7

1. Cookery (Beans). 2. Cookery (Lentils). 3. Cookery (Tofu).

TX803.B4B42 2000   641.6'565   C00-931299-4

Foreword

Great discoveries are often accidental. If Archimedes hadn't been taking a bath, he wouldn't have devised the basic principle of hydrostatics. And Isaac Newton, had he not been in the path of a falling apple, might never have given us the theory of gravity. Christopher Columbus, too, was no stranger to chance: He set sail for Cathay in search of valuable spices such as cinnamon and cloves; instead, he landed in the New World, where he discovered allspice, cocoa — and the haricot bean.

Not that beans, as such, were new to European cooks. Beans (and their botanical relation, lentils) had been cultivated by the ancient Egyptians, the Greeks and the Romans, among others, and both made their way across Europe as civilization moved north and west. In Columbus's time, Europe's favorite bean was the broad (or fava) bean. Yet the haricot bean was something quite new, and further enriched the Europeans' knowledge of that category of food we know today as legumes, which includes chickpeas, beans, soybeans and lentils.

Today legumes remain one of the world's most widely consumed and versatile foods. But the fact is that in North America, at least, beans and lentils (and soybean-derived relative, tofu) have something of an image problem. Often perceived as difficult to cook, they have also acquired a reputation for being, well, pretty bland and unexciting. However, as the recipes in this book demonstrate, nothing could be further from the truth.

The fact is that legumes and tofu are key ingredients in signature dishes of countries around the world. What would Italy be without *pasta e fagioli*, the Middle East without hummus, India without *dal*, Greece without *fassolada*, Mexico without *frijoles refritos* or France without cassoulet? Who could imagine oriental cuisine without the ubiquitous tofu, which is sliced, diced, stuffed and stir-fried, to be eaten with equal gusto in street bazaars and the most elegant restaurants? And how many North Americans could live without the occasional feast of chili or old-fashioned baked beans?

At Robert Rose, we've published a number of cookbooks over the years that contain some absolutely outstanding bean, lentil and tofu dishes. So it only seemed natural that we should ask our authors to pool their best dishes in a single volume. And here it is: *The Beans, Lentils and Tofu Gourmet*. Quite simply, we think it's the best collection of its kind.

These recipes offer a spectacular variety of tastes, textures and cooking styles. Yet they are also relatively quick and easy to prepare, and use ingredients that can be found in most supermarkets. We've also included 16 pages of beautiful color photographs to provide additional inspiration, as well as an introduction to the essentials of storing, cooking — and enjoying! — beans, lentils and tofu.

We invite you to discover the rich variety of dishes that await you in this book. Like Columbus, you may be surprised by what you find.

– *The Editors of Robert Rose*

All About Beans, Lentils and Tofu

Beans and **lentils** are delicious hot or cold, are visually appealing and come in many different shapes, sizes and colors — including yellow chickpeas, red or white kidney beans, and multi-colored lentils. They are highly adaptable, combining well with a wide variety of flavors and foods, running the gamut from graceful and elegant (LENTIL AND PANCETTA ANTIPASTO, see page 23) to rib-sticking hearty (WAGON BOSS CHILI, see page 94). Legumes can make inspiring appetizers (BLACK BEAN AND ROASTED GARLIC SPREAD, see page 22), the most stylish of salads, (LENTIL AND BEET SALAD, see page 74), distinctive soups (PUMPKIN AND WHITE BEAN SOUP, see page 48) and delicious entrées (SALMON OVER WHITE-AND-BLACK BEAN SALSA, see page 124). Better still, they are inexpensive and highly nutritious. In fact, if it weren't for dried beans and lentils, many of our pioneer ancestors wouldn't have survived. Because they were easy to store, legumes were a crucial source of nutrition for an age that lacked refrigeration, as well as seasonal supplies of fresh fruit and vegetables.

Tofu, a curd made from soybeans, was first used in China around 200 BC. Today, it is a dietary staple throughout Asia where it is often combined with meat or fish and served stuffed or as part of a stir-fry. Although tofu is quite bland, it has a remarkable ability to soak up flavors and makes an excellent background for robust sauces. Tofu is actually a great convenience food and you should learn to think of it as an ingredient rather than a meal in itself.

There are three main types of tofu. *Firm tofu* is dense, solid and holds its shape in stir-fries and soups or under the broiler and on the grill; it is higher in protein, fat and calcium than other varieties. *Soft tofu* works best when blended or mashed into dishes, and *silken tofu* is a creamy custard-like product that works well puréed. Silken tofu is particularly good for dips and sauces.

Here are some ideas for using tofu in everyday dishes:

- For any recipe that calls for cream, mayonnaise, sour cream, cream cheese or ricotta, replace half the amount with silken tofu.
- Make a topping for baked potatoes. Combine 1/2 cup (125 mL) silken tofu with 1/2 cup (125 mL) low-fat sour cream and 1/4 cup (50 mL) chopped green onions or chives.
- Add pieces of firm tofu to chili, stews, casseroles or soups.

Whatever recipes you choose to make from this book, introducing more tofu to your diet will add variety and nutrition to your meal planning. And, with inventive dishes like MALAY VEGETABLE STUFFED FRIED BEAN CURD WITH SPICY SWEET-AND-SOUR PEANUT SAUCE (page 20) or CHICKPEA TOFU STEW (page 100), you'll never think tofu is boring again.

NUTRITION FACTS

Beans and lentils. Although the benefits vary between different types, legumes share some common nutritional characteristics. All are a rich source of B-vitamins, calcium, iron, phosphorous, potassium and zinc. They are also high in folate — a B-vitamin that plays a role in cell formation and is particularly beneficial for pregnant women, since it reduces the risk of neural tube defects in embryos.

Legumes are also an excellent source of low-fat *protein*. A diet rich in beans and lentils can help to provide necessary protein without the added cholesterol and fat contained in meat. Today, more and more people are adopting a vegetarian lifestyle. As a rich source of vegetable protein, legumes are an ideal staple for vegetarian diets. It should be noted, however, that they do not contain the entire range of essential amino acids that allows them to be classified as a "complete" protein. Consequently, strict vegetarians should ensure they eat adequate amounts of grains and cereals, seeds and nuts, dairy products and eggs in addition to legumes.

Clinical studies have shown repeatedly the benefits of a diet that is *high in fiber* and *low in fat* — which, unfortunately, is pretty much the antithesis of how most North Americans eat. Consuming adequate amounts of fiber and cutting down on fat can reduce the chances of getting cancer and heart disease, or suffering from a stroke. Not only does fiber help to promote good bowel functioning and lower blood cholesterol levels, it can also help to control blood sugar levels in people with diabetes. Moreover, a lack of dietary fiber has been linked to colon cancer, a leading cause of death in North America.

Given that nutritionists recommend consuming 25 to 35 grams of fiber a day, a diet rich in legumes goes a long way towards meeting this goal. Although the quantity of dietary fiber varies with different types of legume, 1 cup [250 mL] cooked legumes generally provides one-third of the daily requirement.

With so many healthful properties, legumes are particularly beneficial for people on special diets. For instance, they are *low in sodium* — good news for people with high blood pressure, problems with fluid retention or kidney and liver disease. They are also a good source of nutrition for people on *gluten-free* or iron-fortified diets. There is also evidence to suggest that legumes are a natural appetite suppressant; because they are digested slowly and cause a low, sustained increase in blood sugar, eating legumes can delay the onset of hunger and make it easier to control eating.

Tofu. Recently, tofu has been creating quite a stir among nutritionists and health professionals because of its potential health benefits. In addition to being a source of high-grade *protein* — comparable to meat in both quality and digestibility — tofu is a good source of *B-vitamins*, *potassium* and *iron*. It also contains *linoleic and oleic acids,* as well as *lecithin*, all of which are believed to inhibit growth of cholesterol on the walls of blood vessels. When *calcium* is used as the curdling agent, tofu is an excellent source of that mineral as well. For example, a 1/2-cup [125 mL] serving of regular tofu made with calcium sulphate contains 430 mg of calcium; that's over 40% of the recommended daily intake for adults. Tofu also contains essential *amino acids* that aid in digestion and the utilization of other foods.

Like soybeans, tofu is also a rich source of special compounds called *isoflavones*. (Rich in soy protein, one half cup [125 mL] tofu contains 30 to 50 milligrams of isoflavones.) Over the past 10 years a growing body of research has indicated that isoflavones are beneficial in fighting a wide range of diseases, including cancer, heart disease and osteoporosis. In fact, the evidence linking soy protein with health is so compelling that in 1999 the FDA agreed that manufacturers could claim that by lowering blood cholesterol levels, soy protein reduced the risk of coronary heart disease. Lowering cholesterol levels requires that 25 g soy protein be added daily to a diet already low in saturated fat and cholesterol.

Given such healthful benefits, it's not surprising that more and more people have been introducing soy into their diets. Yet many people are still foregoing soy protein as a source of isoflavones, relying upon supplements instead. This concerns scientists who see supplements as pharmacological compounds, not foods, and who suspect that taking isoflavone supplements may have long-term health risks. Although the evidence is not yet in, there is little doubt that the safest strategy is to consume isoflavones as part of a whole food such as tofu, rather than as a supplement.

THE "GAS PROBLEM"

While a high-fiber diet is beneficial to health, flatulence may be an undesirable side effect. Fortunately, there are techniques for mitigating this problem. Introducing legumes into your diet by eating more easily digested varieties, such as split peas and lentils, and gradually increasing the quantities so your body can adapt over time is one way to reduce abdominal discomfort. You should also avoid eating legumes with other gas-producing vegetables such as cabbage, cauliflower, broccoli and Brussels sprouts. Indian cooks, who have been making *dal* for centuries, know a thing or two about limiting the potential consequences of eating legumes. They often season their lentils with spices that aid digestion, such as ginger root or fennel. Another technique is to add a pinch of baking soda to the water in which dried legumes are soaked. Finally, a digestive enzyme such as Beano can help to break down the fiber, making it easier to digest.

BUYING AND STORING LEGUMES AND TOFU

Dried beans and lentils can be purchased in various package sizes at most supermarkets or from bulk-food stores. They should be stored in a dry, airtight container at room temperature. Since they lose their moisture over time, they are best used within a year. Not only do old beans take longer to soak and to cook, they are likely to be tougher than beans that have been stored for only a few months.

Once cooked, legumes should be covered and stored in the refrigerator where they will keep for 4 or 5 days. Cooked legumes can also be frozen. Packaged in an airtight, freezer-friendly container, they will keep frozen for up to 6 months.

Tofu is sold in water-filled tubs or vacuum packs and can be found in the produce or dairy section of supermarkets. Since it has a limited shelf life, check the "best before" date on the package. After the package has been opened, drain the liquid, place any unused portions in a bowl and cover with fresh cold water. Store, covered, in the refrigerator. Tofu will keep for 1 week if the water is changed daily. If it develops a sour smell, throw it out.

COOKED VS. CANNED LEGUMES

The same variety of cooked dried legumes can be substituted for canned legumes in any of the recipes in this book. When cooking dried beans and lentils, bear in mind that they will more than double in size after cooking. Because their sizes and shapes vary so dramatically, it's difficult to give exact ratios between uncooked and cooked quantities of legumes, but you're fairly safe using 1 cup [250 mL] uncooked legumes in a recipe that requires 2 cups [500 mL] cooked. (Just remember to soak, when appropriate, and cook according to the following directions before adding them to your recipe.)

Canned beans are a quick and easy substitute for cooked dried beans. For 2 cups [500 mL] cooked beans, use a standard 19-oz [540 mL] can. Rinse well under cold running water before adding to your recipe.

COOKING LEGUMES

Before using dried beans and lentils, spread them out on a piece of paper or a large platter and sort through to remove any that are damaged or discolored, as well as any foreign matter. This is particularly important for those purchased in bulk.

If using dried beans, they will need to be soaked before cooking, using one of the methods described below.

Lentils and split peas, on the other hand, usually do not need to be pre-soaked. In a colander or sieve, rinse under cold water until it runs clear and the legumes are thoroughly washed. Depending on the type, their cooking time varies from 10 minutes for red, pink and French lentils to 45 minutes for split peas. To ensure proper cooking time, follow the recipes in this book.

Stove-top method

When cooking dried beans, the first step is to replace the water that has been lost in the drying process. This can be done by either of two methods. The beans can be soaked overnight (beans cooked by this method cook in less time and keep their shape better) or they can be brought to a boil then left to sit for an hour. In both cases, use 3 parts water to 1 part beans by volume.

Once the beans are in the cooking pot, you can start the seasoning process. Don't add salt until the end of the cooking time or the beans will become tough. You can, however, embellish their flavor while they cook by adding enhancements such as a clove-studded onion, some garlic, bay leaves or a *bouquet garni* made of parsley, celery, thyme and bay leaf tied together in a piece of cheesecloth.

You can help to reduce the incidence of gas by following these techniques in the cooking process. First, rinse dried beans under cold running water before soaking. Then add a good pinch of baking soda to the soaking water. After soaking, drain the beans and rinse again. Then simmer in fresh water, (3 parts water to 1 part beans) as slowly as possible until the beans are tender. This usually takes 1 to 2 hours or just until the skin breaks easily.

Microwave method

Pre-Soak. In a 12-cup [3 L] microwavable bowl, combine 3 cups [750 mL] hot water with 1 cup [250 mL] dried beans. Cover tightly with plastic wrap. Microwave on High for 10 to 15 minutes. Set aside for an hour. Drain and rinse under cold water. Use in recipe or cook as described below.

Cooking. In a microwavable bowl, combine soaked, drained beans with 4 cups [1 L] hot water. Cover tightly with plastic wrap and microwave on High for 35 min. Allow to rest, covered, for an additional 20 minutes.

Slow-cooker method

Pre-Soak. In a colander rinse dried beans thoroughly under cold running water. In a large pot or bowl, combine 1 part beans with 3 parts water and a pinch of baking soda. Soak overnight or bring to a boil and allow to sit for 1 hour. Drain, rinse thoroughly under cold running water, and cook as described below.

Cooking. In a slow cooker, combine 2 cups [500 mL] pre-soaked beans and 6 cups [1.5 L] water. Season with garlic, bay leaves, or a *bouquet garni* made from your favorite herbs tied together in cheesecloth, if desired. Cook on Low for 8 to 10 hours. The beans are now ready to be used in your favorite recipe.

The Beans, Lentils and Tofu Gourmet

Contributing Authors

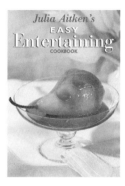

Julia Aitken, author of the *Easy Entertaining Cookbook*, is a leading food writer and cookbook author with more than 20 years of experience. Currently food editor of *Elm Street* magazine, her guests rarely cancel when she entertains.

In the *Easy Entertaining Cookbook,* Julia provides over 125 elegant-but-easy recipes, helpful tips and kitchen wisdom, as well as refreshingly frank advice on how to ensure a successful dinner party. (Rule #1: Only invite people you like.) Put that together with a great selection of flavorful dishes and you've got the perfect recipe for years of relaxed, enjoyable entertaining. Recipes from this book are found on pages 23, 38, 69 and 180.

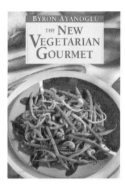

Byron Ayanoglu, author of *The New Vegetarian Gourmet* and *Simply Mediterranean Cooking*, has devoted his life to wonderful food. He has worked as a restaurant critic, as Mick Jagger's personal chef and is Robert de Niro's favorite movie-set caterer.

In *The New Vegetarian Gourmet*, you can create fast and easy culinary magic with over 120 exquisite vegetarian recipes. Here you'll find sumptuous flavors and textures that will delight vegetarians and non-vegetarians alike. Better yet, the recipes are remarkably easy to prepare. This book sets the standard for kitchens where good health and good-tasting food are equally important. Recipes from this book are found on pages 42, 72, 100, 102, 138, 152, 164, 165, 168, 170 and 171.

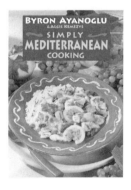

With *Simply Mediterranean Cooking*, discover food that transports you to a world of azure skies, olive groves and fresh sea breezes. That's the essence of Mediterranean cooking — and it's what you'll find in this book. This is food that begs to be tasted. And it's as delicious as it is easy to prepare. In fact, this may be the only Mediterranean cookbook you'll ever need. The book was written with the help of Algis Kemezys, Byron's longtime sous chef and an internationally exhibited photographic artist. Recipes from this book are found on pages 19, 78, 80, 82, 84, 112, 114, 128, 130 and 132.

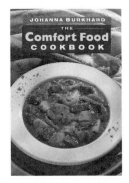

Johanna Burkhard, author of *The Comfort Food Cookbook* and *Fast & Easy Cooking*, is one of Canada's leading food writers. A former food columnist at the *Montreal Gazette*, she has been a regular contributor for over a decade to many national magazines, including *Canadian Living*, *Homemaker's*, *Wine Tidings* and *Elm Street*.

The Comfort Food Cookbook is all about food that's simply, satisfyingly delicious. That's comfort food — and here's a book that features over 125 fast, easy-to-prepare recipes for the most comforting dishes you've ever tasted. A portion of the proceeds from each sale goes to the Children's Miracle Network. Recipes from this book are found on pages 25, 67, 91, 92 and 109.

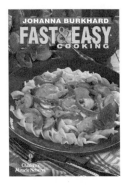

Fast & Easy Cooking. Sure, you'd like to give your family a delicious, home-cooked meal. But at the end of a long day, who's got the time? You do! With *Fast & Easy Cooking*, you'll discover that there really is an alternative to commercially prepared "convenience foods." Here are over 100 recipes, specially designed for today's families, along with hundreds of tips that will make meal preparation faster and easier. Recipes from this book are found on pages 26, 39, 47, 86, 93, 134 and 149.

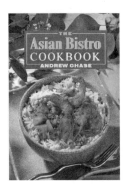

Andrew Chase, author of *The Asian Bistro Cookbook*, was educated at Columbia University in New York and National Taiwan University in Taipei, subsequently working in Taipei, Hong Kong, Manila and Shanghai. Since 1988, he has owned and worked as chef at a number of restaurants in the U.S. and Canada, including Café Asia, Berkeley Café, and Youki Asian Bar and Bistro.

The Asian Bistro Cookbook opens up exciting new territory for anyone who loves the distinctive flavors of Asian cooking. Taste the best of China, Japan and Thailand — plus the Philippines, Korea, Vietnam, Indonesia and Taiwan. These recipes are unusual, delicious and, best of all, amazingly simple to prepare. Recipes from this book are found on pages 20, 40, 106, 160, 161 and 162.

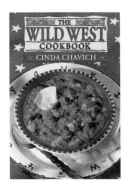

Cinda Chavich, author of *The Wild West Cookbook*, is food editor of the Calgary Herald and is one of the top food writers in western Canada. She is a confirmed westerner who loves all things Western — from food to lifestyle.

With *The Wild West Cookbook* you can discover for yourself the flavorful, stick-to-your-ribs cooking that sustained generations of ranch hands from Abilene to Alberta. Here you'll find over 120 easy-to-prepare recipes, plus a rich selection of contemporary cowboy images and fascinating historical anecdotes that will enhance your appreciation of this timeless cuisine. Recipes from this book are found on pages 31, 32, 34, 49, 50, 51, 74, 76, 87, 88, 94, 95, 96, 98, 104, 118 and 178.

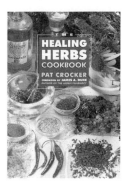

Pat Crocker, author of *The Healing Herbs Cookbook*, is a culinary herbalist and professional home economist with more than 25 years experience. She has written about the use of herbs in cooking for many newspapers and magazines. She also gives lectures and conducts walking tours of her teaching herb gardens.

The Healing Herbs Cookbook. Alternative therapies are a growing trend, and many scientific studies now point to the health benefits of herbs used in foods. The bestselling *Healing Herbs Cookbook* contains more than 100 recipes featuring one or more healing herbs. In addition to great recipes, this book provides useful information on preserving and cooking with herbs. A list of herbal sources, glossary and herb-specific recipe index are also included. This is the ideal book for people who want to bring the benefits of healing herbs into the kitchen. Recipes from this book are found on pages 22, 64, 99, 142, 146 and 148.

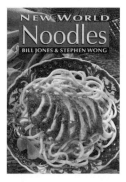

Bill Jones and Stephen Wong, co-authors of *New World Noodles* and *New World Chinese Cooking*. Bill is a food consultant who works with Vancouver-area restaurants such as Sooke Harbour House. He also promotes B.C. food products in China and has wide-ranging experience in Asian and North American cuisine. Stephen is a Vancouver-based restaurant consultant and food writer. He is the author of a number of successful cookbooks.

New World Noodles. Everyone loves the simplicity of pasta. And now there's something even better. *New World Noodles* brings a fresh approach to mealtime, blending Eastern and Western flavors to give you over 100 tantalizing dishes. Best of all, these recipes are easy to make and can be prepared with widely available ingredients. So move over pasta — here come the noodles! Recipes from this book are found on page 44.

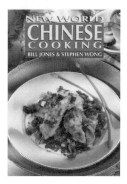

New World Chinese Cooking. Take the best of Chinese cooking and put it together with an imaginative variety of North American ingredients. What have you got? The next step in Chinese cookbooks — *New World Chinese Cooking*. Don't mistake this for old-style Chinese cooking. It's easy, accessible and delicious. Recipes from this book are found on pages 46, 108, 122, 172 and 173.

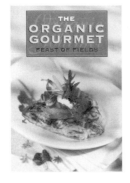

Tracy Kett, who compiled and edited *The Organic Gourmet*, is a Toronto-based writer and caterer who has provided editorial services for a number of national magazines, newspapers and environmental groups. She has a long-standing interest in promoting organic agriculture for a healthier planet and society.

The Organic Gourmet. In recent years more and more people have come to appreciate the health and flavor benefits of organic foods. Now, with *The Organic Gourmet*, you get over 100 recipes that show just how sensationally delicious organic food can be. Also included is a wealth of cooking tips and background information, plus a comprehensive reference to organic ingredients, standards and sources. Recipes from this book are found on pages 55 and 60.

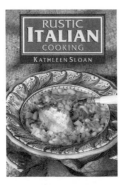

Kathleen Sloan, author of *Rustic Italian Cooking* and *The Global Grill*, is an established food writer whose work has appeared in a variety of newspapers and magazines, including *The Globe and Mail*, *The Toronto Star*, *Chatelaine*, *Flare*, *Homemaker's*, *Canadian House and Home* and *Wine Tidings*.

Rustic Italian Cooking is all about food the way it has been enjoyed in Italy for centuries — simple, unpretentious, hearty and delicious. This is real Italian cooking, the kind that you'll find only by venturing into the countryside. With *Rustic Italian Cooking*, you can experience all the best regional cuisine that Italy has to offer. Unusual and appetizing, these dishes are above all simple, accessible and easy to prepare. Recipes from this book are found on pages 18, 52, 53, 54, 56, 58, 75, 110, 116, 121, 175, 176 and 177.

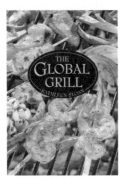

The Global Grill. From the time that our primitive ancestors first prepared food over an open flame, the grill has occupied a special place in cooking traditions around the world. With over 120 recipes drawn from every continent, *The Global Grill* takes you on a uniquely international tour of grilled food. For anyone who loves grilling, this book serves up a world of eating pleasure. Recipes from this book are found on pages 90, 166 and 167.

Appetizers

Fagioli bianchi alla menta
White bean with mint

Blanch mint and parsley leaves in boiling water for 10 seconds; remove immediately and drain.

This spread is wonderful served on crostini. Italian for "little toasts", crostini are thin slices of bread that are toasted and, most often, brushed with a little olive oil.

1 cup	whole mint leaves, blanched and drained	250 mL
1 cup	whole flat-leaf parsley leaves, blanched and drained	250 mL
4	cloves garlic, peeled	4
1 1/2 cups	cooked cannellini beans (white kidney beans)	375 mL
2 tbsp	extra virgin olive oil	25 mL
	Salt and freshly ground black pepper	

1. In a food processor, combine mint, parsley and garlic; process until finely chopped. Add beans; process for 1 minute or until well-combined, scraping down sides of bowl at halfway point. Add oil; process until smooth. Season to taste with salt and pepper.

Lentils with spicy sausage

Serves 4 to 6 as an appetizer or 3 to 4 as a main course

North Americans are finally acknowledging the lowly lentil for the miracle food that it is. Not only total protein nutrition, but also delicious and endlessly adaptable, with a slew of tasty recipes to choose from. Here's a winter-type lentil that can make either for a good entrée on its own, or a hearty main course served with boiled potato and green salad. The butter enhancement is optional if it offends the calorie-wise, but it will obviously add a welcome richness to the proceedings.

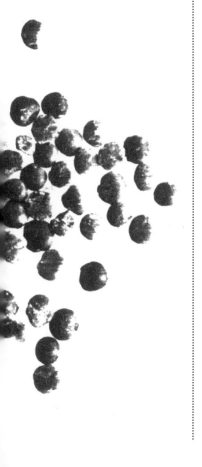

1 cup	green lentils	250 mL
4 cups	boiling water	1 L
4 or 5	cloves garlic, sliced	4 or 5
1	bay leaf	1
1/2 tsp	dried thyme	2 mL
1/4 tsp	freshly ground black pepper	1 mL
8 oz	spicy sausage (merguez, chorizo or spicy Italian)	250 g
1/2 cup	sliced onions	125 mL
1 tbsp	butter (optional)	15 mL
1 tsp	white wine vinegar	5 mL
	Salt to taste	
	Several sprigs fresh parsley, chopped	

1. In a pot soak lentils in 2 cups (500 mL) of the boiling water for 20 minutes. (Lentils will swell up and absorb most of the water.) Add remaining 2 cups (500 mL) boiling water; stir in the garlic, bay leaf, thyme and pepper. Cook, uncovered, over medium heat for 30 minutes, stirring very occasionally. At the end of this period the lentils should be tender but still holding their shape; if too much water has boiled off (there should be enough moisture to give a saucy appearance to the lentils), add 1/2 to 1 cup (125 to 250 mL) more water as needed.

2. Meanwhile, broil sausage and onions for 3 to 4 minutes on each side. (They should not cook through; neither should the onions burn.) Remove and slice sausage into 1/2-inch (1 cm) pieces. Set aside sausage and onions together.

3. When the lentils are done, transfer to an ovenproof dish. Add butter (if using), vinegar and salt. Stir to mix. Add sausage and onions; stir until well distributed. Bake uncovered in a preheated 400° F (200° C) oven for 30 minutes. Serve immediately garnished with chopped fresh parsley.

Malay vegetable-stuffed fried bean curd with spicy sweet-and-sour peanut sauce

Serves 4

A refreshing first course, this dish exemplifies the creative mix of Malaysian cuisine. The relatively bland Chinese ingredient, bean curd, is stuffed with fresh, crunchy vegetables and topped with a spicy sweet-and-sour peanut sauce of obvious Southeast Asian origin, except that it relies on soya sauce (or fermented soybeans) — again, Chinese. By now, Chinese culinary influences — as well as Indian and, to some extent, European — have blended so long with the indigenous Malay cuisine that a recipe such as this one is essentially Malaysian.

Use your imagination in varying the vegetables used for the stuffing; it can make delicious use of leftover produce. Some suitable vegetables include string or long beans, pea pods (snow peas), jicama, chayote squash, Napa cabbage, sweet potato and zucchini.

1 lb	firm tofu (bean curd)	500 g
1/3 cup	vegetable oil	75 mL
1/4 cup	carrot julienne	50 mL
1/2 cup	bean sprouts	125 mL
1/2 cup	seeded cucumber julienne	125 mL
2 tbsp	red bell pepper julienne	25 mL
1/2 cup	raw peanuts *or* commercially dry-roasted peanuts	125 mL
3 to 6	finely chopped red chilies, preferably bird-eye chilies	3 to 6
1 1/2 tsp	minced garlic	7 mL
1 tbsp	tamarind paste *or* 2 tsp (10 mL) vinegar *or* 1 tbsp (15 mL) lime or lemon juice	15 mL
2 tbsp	palm sugar *or* light brown sugar	25 mL
2 1/2 tsp	soya sauce	12 mL

1. Cut tofu into 4 equal parts. Lay cakes on a plate and weight with a flat-bottomed plate to press out excess water; leave for 1 hour. Pat cakes dry. In a nonstick skillet, heat oil over medium-high heat; cook cakes until golden and crispy, about 5 minutes per side.

2. Blanch carrots in boiling water until almost tender; rinse in cold water. Blanch bean sprouts for 5 seconds; rinse in cold water. Mix together carrots, bean sprouts, cucumber and red pepper; set aside.

3. In a dry pan, toast raw peanuts over medium heat until golden. Grind peanuts until fine. Pound the chilies and garlic into a paste (or chop together until very fine with chili seeds broken up completely). Mix tamarind paste with 2 tbsp (25 mL) boiling water and work until pulp is completely dissolved and loosened from the seeds; strain liquid and mix with sugar and soya sauce (if using vinegar or citrus juice, stir together with 1 tbsp [15 mL] water, sugar and soya sauce). When sugar is dissolved, stir in chili and garlic paste. Stir in enough ground peanuts to make a thick sauce.

4. Cut each tofu cake in half horizontally. Remove top halves; top bottom pieces with vegetable mixture and replace top pieces. Cut each stuffed cake in half or in quarters from corner to corner. Spoon sauce over cakes and serve.

Black bean and roasted garlic spread

Tip

Black turtle beans give a smooth texture to this healing spread.

Variations

Substitute: Red wine or healing vinegar for balsamic vinegar.

PREHEAT OVEN TO 375° F (190° C)
SMALL CASSEROLE DISH, WITH LID

4	whole garlic heads	4
1/2 tbsp	olive oil	7 mL
1	can (19 oz [540 mL]) black beans	1
1 tbsp	olive oil	15 mL
2 tsp	balsamic vinegar	10 mL

1. Slice 1/4 inch (5 mm) off the top of each garlic head. Remove outer loose skin. Place each head cut-side up in casserole dish. Drizzle with 1/2 tbsp (7 mL) oil. Cover and bake in preheated oven for 40 to 45 minutes or until cloves are very soft. Remove from oven and allow to cool.

2. Meanwhile, place black beans in a food processor or blender. When garlic is cool enough to handle, squeeze cloves from heads into the food processor. Process until smooth. With the motor running, add olive oil and vinegar; process until combined. If desired, season to taste with salt and pepper. Store in the refrigerator for up to 3 days.

Lentil and pancetta antipasto

Serves 6

Pancetta is Italian bacon cured with nutmeg, cinnamon or cloves to give it a distinctive flavor. If pancetta is unavailable, regular bacon can be substituted, but the flavor won't be as authentically Italian.

Kitchen Wisdom
For a colorful antipasti platter to serve as a sit-down appetizer, spoon this salad onto a platter, along with antipasto, a couple of tomatoes cut into wedges, a selection of olives and some sliced mozzarella or bocconcini cheese.

Make Ahead
Antipasto can be refrigerated, covered, for up to 24 hours. Let stand at room temperature for 30 minutes before serving.

1 cup	green lentils	250 mL
4	sprigs fresh oregano or marjoram	4
2 oz	pancetta, chopped	50 g
2	stalks celery, finely chopped	2
Half	medium red onion, finely chopped	Half
1/4 cup	chopped fresh Italian flat-leafed parsley	50 mL
1	clove garlic, minced	1
2 tbsp	olive oil	25 mL
1 tbsp	chopped fresh oregano or marjoram	15 mL
1 tbsp	red wine vinegar	15 mL
1/2 tsp	black pepper	2 mL
1/4 tsp	salt	1 mL

1. Rinse lentils under running water, picking them over and discarding any grit. Drain well. Bring a medium saucepan of water to boil over high heat. Add lentils and oregano sprigs; cook, uncovered, for 15 to 20 minutes or until lentils are tender but still firm. Drain well, discarding oregano; transfer lentils to a large serving bowl.

2. In a small heavy skillet, cook pancetta over medium-high heat for 2 to 3 minutes or until just starting to crisp. With a slotted spoon, remove pancetta from skillet; drain on a paper-towel-lined plate.

3. Add pancetta, celery, onion, parsley and garlic to lentils; toss well. Sprinkle with oil, oregano, vinegar, pepper and salt; toss well. If desired, season to taste with additional salt and pepper. Serve at room temperature.

Serves 4 to 6 or
makes 1 cup (250 mL)

Hummus
Chickpea sauce

Variation
Herbs such as coriander,
Thai basil or mint can be
added to the vegetables for
extra flavor. Add about 1 tbsp
(15 mL) fine julienne.

Tip
Tahini is a Middle Eastern
condiment found in the
specialty section of some
supermarkets. If unavailable,
use peanut butter.

Surround the dip with
crackers, fresh vegetable
sticks or pita bread pieces.

Make Ahead
Prepare dip up to a day
before. Stir just before serving and garnish with parsley.

1/4 cup	water	50 mL
1 cup	drained canned chickpeas	250 mL
3/4 tsp	crushed garlic	4 mL
2 tbsp	lemon juice	25 mL
4 tsp	olive oil	20 mL
1/4 cup	tahini	50 mL
1 tbsp	chopped fresh parsley	15 mL

1. In a food processor, combine water, chickpeas, garlic,
lemon juice, oil and tahini; process until creamy and
smooth.

2. Transfer to serving dish; sprinkle with parsley.

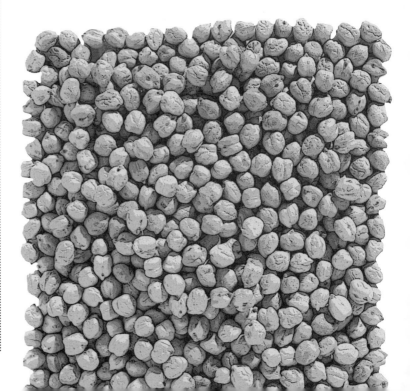

Serves 4

Cheese and salsa quesadillas

Here's my modern rendition of grilled cheese: thin flour tortillas replace sliced bread, mozzarella substitutes for processed cheese and chunky salsa stands in for the ketchup. And the beans? They're optional, but make a wholesome addition.

Tip

I often serve these warm cheesy wedges with soup for an easy dinner. They're also great as a snack that both kids and grownups applaud.

Use mild salsa to appease those with timid taste buds, but add a dash of hot pepper sauce to the filling for those who like a burst of heat.

1/2 cup	prepared salsa, plus additional for serving	125 mL
4	flour tortillas (8-inch [20 cm] size)	4
1 cup	canned black or pinto beans, rinsed and drained well	250 mL
1 cup	shredded mozzarella, Monterey Jack or Cheddar cheese	250 mL

1. Spread 2 tbsp (25 mL) salsa on one-half of each tortilla. Sprinkle with 1/4 cup (50 mL) each of the beans and the cheese. Fold tortillas over and press down lightly.

2. Heat a large nonstick skillet over medium heat; cook tortillas, 2 at a time, pressing down lightly with the back of a metal spatula, for about 2 minutes per side, until lightly toasted and cheese is melted. Or, place directly on barbecue grill over medium heat until lightly toasted on both sides.

3. Cut into wedges and serve warm with additional salsa, if desired.

Always popular layered bean dip

Serves 8

Variations of the popular bean dip have been making the party circuit in recent years. Here's my updated version. It has an oregano/bean base, a creamy jalapeño cheese layer and a vibrant fresh topping of tomatoes, olives and coriander.

Tip
To make pita crisps, separate 3 (7-inch [18 cm]) thin pitas into rounds. Cut into 8 wedges each. Place in single layer on 2 baking sheets: bake in 350° F (180° C) oven for 8 to 10 minutes or until crisp and lightly toasted. Transfer to a rack to cool. Can be prepared up to a week ahead and stored in an airtight container or frozen.

8-INCH (20 CM) SHALLOW ROUND SERVING DISH OR PIE PLATE

1	can (19 oz [540 mL]) red kidney beans or black beans, rinsed and drained	1
1	clove garlic, minced	1
1 tsp	dried oregano	5 mL
1/2 tsp	ground cumin	2 mL
1 cup	shredded Monterey Jack or Cheddar cheese	250 mL
3/4 cup	light sour cream	175 mL
1 tbsp	minced pickled jalapeño peppers	15 mL
2	tomatoes, seeded and finely diced	2
1	Haas avocado, peeled and diced (optional)	1
2	green onions	2
1/3 cup	sliced black olives	75 mL
1/3 cup	chopped fresh coriander or parsley	75 mL

1. In a food processor, combine beans, garlic, oregano, cumin and 1 tbsp (15 mL) water; process until smooth. Spread in serving dish.

2. In a bowl combine cheese, sour cream and jalapeño peppers. Spread over bean layer. (Can be assembled earlier in day; cover and refrigerate.)

3. Just before serving, sprinkle with tomatoes, avocado (if using), green onions, olives and coriander. Serve with pita crisps (see note, at left).

Bean and cheese tortilla slices

Serves 4 to 6

Tip
Substitute black or white kidney beans for the red kidney beans.

Serve as an appetizer or as a side dish.

For a more decorative look, add 1 lettuce leaf to top of filling before rolling.

Make Ahead
Prepare up to 1 day in advance; cut just before serving.

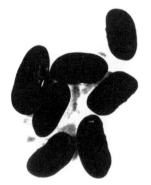

1 cup	canned red kidney beans, rinsed and drained	250 mL
1 tbsp	freshly squeezed lemon juice	15 mL
1/2 tsp	chili powder	2 mL
1/2 tsp	minced garlic	2 mL
3/4 cup	5% smooth ricotta cheese	175 mL
3 tbsp	chopped green onions	45 mL
3 tbsp	chopped fresh coriander	45 mL
2 tbsp	light sour cream	25 mL
1 tbsp	light mayonnaise	15 mL
4	small 6-inch (15 cm) flour tortillas	4

1. In a food processor or with a fork in a bowl, mash together beans, lemon juice, chili powder and garlic. In a separate bowl, combine ricotta cheese, green onions, coriander, sour cream and mayonnaise; stir until well mixed.
2. Divide ricotta mixture among tortillas and spread over surface. Top with bean mixture. Roll tightly, cover and chill for 30 minutes.
3. Cut each roll into 6 pieces and serve.

Serves 6 to 8

Tofu and chickpea garlic dip

Tip
Tofu combined with beans, such as the chickpeas used here, gives the dip a butter-like texture.

Be sure to buy soft (silken) tofu to ensure a creamy dip. Firm or pressed tofu will result in a granular texture.

Tahini is a sesame paste found in the international section of grocery stores. If you can't find it, try using smooth peanut butter instead.

Make Ahead
Prepare up to 1 day in advance. Mix before serving.

1 cup	canned chickpeas, rinsed and drained	250 mL
8 oz	soft (silken) tofu, drained	250 g
2 tbsp	tahini	25 mL
2 tbsp	freshly squeezed lemon juice	25 mL
1 tsp	minced garlic	5 mL
1/4 cup	chopped fresh dill (or 1 tsp [5 mL] dried)	50 mL
1/4 cup	chopped green onions	50 mL
1/4 cup	chopped green olives	50 mL
1/4 cup	chopped red bell peppers	50 mL
1/4 tsp	freshly ground black pepper	1 mL

1. In a food processor, combine chickpeas, tofu, tahini, lemon juice and garlic; purée. Stir in dill, green onions, olives, red peppers and pepper.
2. Chill. Serve with vegetables, crackers or bread.

White bean and roasted pepper bruschetta

Serves 6 to 8

Tip

Tired of garlic bread? This is a great alternative.

If fresh basil is not available, substitute parsley.

Roast your own red bell peppers or buy water-packed roasted red peppers.

Double recipe and use as a dip.

Make Ahead

Prepare bean mixture up to 1 day in advance.

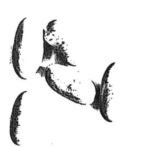

PREHEAT OVEN TO 425° F (220° C)
BAKING SHEET

1 cup	canned white kidney beans, rinsed and drained,	250 mL
1/4 cup	chopped fresh basil (or 1/2 tsp [2 mL] dried)	50 mL
1 1/2 tsp	freshly squeezed lemon juice	7 mL
1/2 tsp	minced garlic	2 mL
1/2 tsp	sesame oil	2 mL
1	baguette or thin French loaf	1
2 tbsp	chopped roasted red peppers	25 mL

1. In a food processor, purée beans, basil, lemon juice, garlic and sesame oil until smooth.

2. Slice baguette into 1-inch (2.5 cm) slices. In a toaster oven or under a preheated broiler, toast until golden; turn and toast opposite side. Spread each slice with approximately 1 1/2 tsp (7 mL) bean mixture. Top with chopped red peppers. Bake in preheated oven for 5 minutes or until warm.

Black and white bean salsa

Serves 6
Makes 3 cups
(750 mL)

Tip
Serve over salad as a side dish.

Great over grains such as couscous or rice.

On non-vegetarian days, try this salsa with fish or chicken.

Make Ahead
Prepare up to 1 day in advance. Mix well before serving.

1 cup	canned black beans, rinsed and drained	250 mL
1 cup	canned navy beans, rinsed and drained	250 mL
1 cup	chopped plum tomatoes	250 mL
1/2 cup	canned corn, drained	125 mL
1/3 cup	chopped fresh coriander	75 mL
1/3 cup	chopped green onions	75 mL
1/3 cup	chopped red bell peppers	75 mL
2 tbsp	freshly squeezed lime juice	25 mL
1 1/2 tbsp	olive oil	22 mL
1 1/2 tsp	chili powder	7 mL
1 tsp	minced garlic	5 mL
	Freshly ground black pepper to taste	

1. In a bowl combine black beans, navy beans, tomatoes, corn, coriander, green onions, red peppers, lime juice, olive oil, chili powder and garlic; mix well. Season to taste with pepper.

Beyond bean dip

Makes about
7 cups (1.75 L)

Although the texture of canned beans is inferior for dishes that call for whole beans, they are simple and fast to use — especially for dips or refried bean dishes. Rinse and drain canned beans before using

Bean Layer

1	can (14 oz [398 mL]) refried beans *or* 1 can (19 oz [540 mL]) pinto beans	1
1/4 cup	sour cream	50 mL
1	jalapeño pepper, seeded and minced	1
1	clove garlic, minced	1
1 tsp	chili powder	5 mL
1/2 tsp	ground cumin	2 mL

Guacamole Layer

2	ripe avocados	2
3 tbsp	lemon juice *or* lime juice	45 mL
3	green onions, minced	3
1 tsp	minced jalapeño pepper	5 mL

Garnish

1 cup	sour cream	250 mL
2	green onions, chopped	2
1	tomato, seeded and chopped	1
1 cup	shredded Cheddar cheese	250 mL
1/2 cup	sliced black olives	125 mL
	Regular and blue corn tortilla chips as accompaniments	

1. If using pinto beans, rinse and drain. Purée beans in food processor; transfer to a bowl. Stir in sour cream, jalapeño, garlic, chili powder and cumin. Set aside.

2. In another bowl, mash avocados with lemon juice. Stir in green onions and jalapeño pepper. Set aside.

3. Spread bean dip in a thin layer over a deep 12-inch (30 cm) platter. Carefully spread guacamole over bean layer. Spread with sour cream, making sure to cover guacamole completely to keep it from darkening. Starting at the outside edge of the plate, make a 2-inch (5 cm) ring of shredded cheese. Inside that ring, sprinkle green onions in a ring. Follow with black olives and finish with a pile of chopped tomato in the center of the plate. Serve with lots of regular and blue corn tortilla chips for scooping.

Black bean nachos

Serves 4

Cowboys may not have eaten nachos at the turn of the century but we certainly consume a lot of corn chips today, a testament to the spread of Tex-Mex cooking throughout the West. Today, nachos have become the national snack in cowboy country. In small-town cafés, rural bars or casual city restaurants, you'll always find nachos to start a meal.

Southern Alberta is home to two of the largest corn chip makers — El Molino Foods and Del Comal Foods.

Use canned beans, rinsed and drained, or cook your own. Start with 1 cup (250 mL) dried black beans.

Salsa

2	plum tomatoes, seeded and chopped	2
1/4 cup	chopped onions	50 mL
1 tbsp	freshly squeezed lime juice	15 mL
1	jalapeño pepper, seeded and minced	1
2 tbsp	minced cilantro	25 mL
1 tbsp	chopped parsley	15 mL
1 tsp	chopped fresh thyme	5 mL
1 tsp	chopped fresh oregano	5 mL
1	green onion, chopped	1

Refried Beans

1 cup	cooked black beans	250 mL
1 tbsp	olive oil	15 mL
1 tbsp	minced garlic	15 mL
2	hot chili peppers, minced	2
1/4 cup	chopped cilantro	50 mL
	Salt to taste	

Guacamole

2	ripe avocados	2
3 tbsp	freshly squeezed lime juice	45 mL
1 tsp	minced garlic	5 mL
1/4 tsp	dried thyme leaves	1 mL
1/4 tsp	dried oregano	1 mL
1	jalapeño pepper, chopped	1
12 cups	combination of yellow and blue tortilla chips	3 L
8 oz	Monterey Jack cheese, shredded	250 g

(Recipe continues...)

CURRY-FRIED TOFU SOUP WITH VEGETABLES AND UDON NOODLES (PAGE 44) ➤

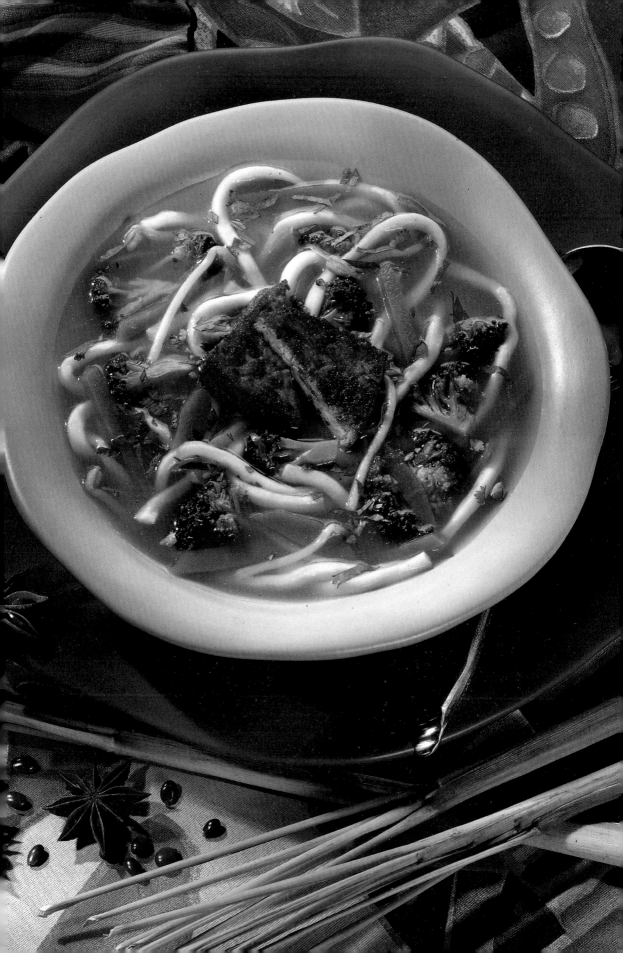

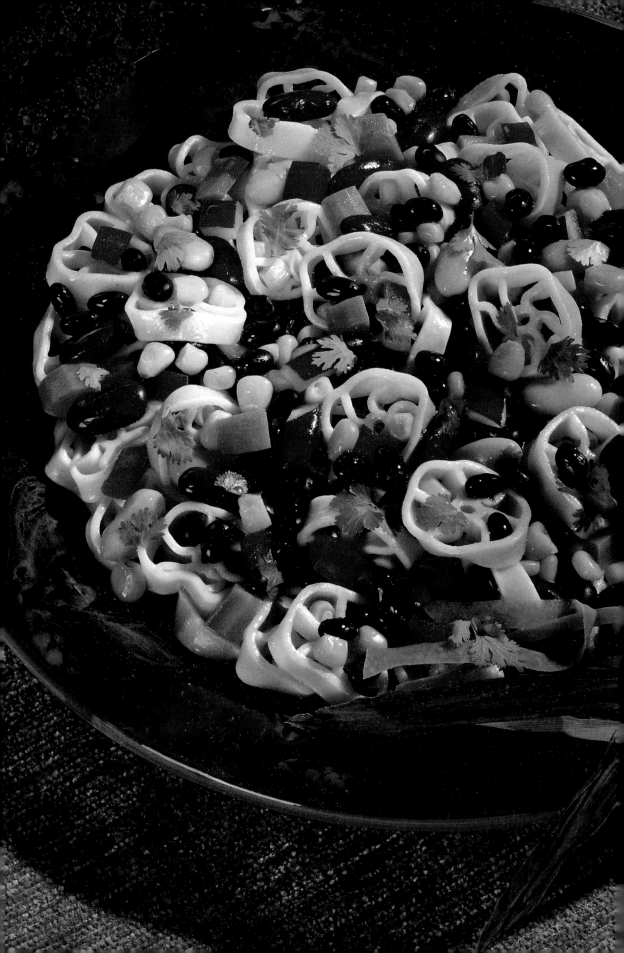

1. **Salsa:** In a bowl, stir together tomatoes, onions, lime juice, jalapeño, cilantro, parsley, thyme, oregano and green onion. Marinate for 1 hour in the refrigerator.

2. **Refried Beans:** Mash beans with a fork or purée in food processor. In a frying pan, heat olive oil over medium heat. Add mashed beans, garlic, chili peppers, and cilantro; cook, stirring, for 3 minutes or until soft and fragrant. Season with salt to taste. Set aside.

3. **Guacamole:** In a bowl and using a fork, mash avocado with lime juice. Stir in garlic, thyme, oregano and jalapeño. Set aside.

4. **Assembly:** Preheat oven to 400° F (200° C). Put tortilla chips on a large ovenproof dish. Distribute refried beans and salsa evenly over chips. Sprinkle with cheese. Bake for 5 minutes or until cheese is melted and dish is hot. Serve with guacamole on the side.

◄ CORN AND THREE-BEAN SALAD (PAGE 66)

**Makes 6 1/2 cups
(1.625 L)**

Use 3 cans (each 19 oz
[540 mL]) black beans or
black-eyed peas, rinsed and
drained, or cook your own
starting with 2 1/2 cups
(625 mL) dried.

Wild west bean caviar with roasted tomatoes

PREHEAT BROILER OR BARBECUE

3	ripe tomatoes	3
2 tbsp	olive oil	25 mL
1/4 cup	red wine vinegar, plus a pinch of granulated sugar *or* balsamic vinegar	50 mL
1 tbsp	lime juice	15mL
3	cloves garlic, minced	3
1/2 tsp	salt	2 mL
6 cups	cooked black beans or black-eyed peas	1.5 L
1/2 cup	chopped red onions	125 mL
1/2 cup	chopped cilantro	125 mL
1	jalapeño pepper, seeded and minced	1
	Corn chips or pita chips	

1. Under the broiler or on the barbecue, cook tomatoes for 10 minutes, turning occasionally, or until charred on all sides. Cool; peel, seed and core. In a food processor, combine tomato flesh, olive oil, vinegar, lime juice, garlic and salt; process until smooth.

2. In a bowl, stir together roasted tomato sauce, beans, red onions, cilantro and jalapeño pepper. Let stand at room temperature for 30 minutes to allow flavors to develop.

3. Serve with corn chips and pita chips for scooping, or serve as a starter salad or side dish.

Soups

Serves 6

Bok choy noodle and tofu chicken soup

2 tsp	sesame oil	10 mL
1 1/2 tsp	minced ginger root	7 mL
1 tsp	crushed garlic	5 mL
2 1/2 cups	chopped bok choy	625 mL
2/3 cup	chopped green onions	150 mL
1/3 cup	chicken stock	75 mL
6 cups	chicken stock	1.5 L
2 tbsp	soya sauce	25 mL
3/4 cup	broken rice vermicelli	175 mL
1/2 cup	chopped snow peas	125 mL
1/2 cup	diced red bell peppers	125 mL
1 cup	firm tofu, cut into small cubes	250 mL

Tip
Napa cabbage, found in the produce section of grocery stores, can replace bok choy.

Spaghettini or capellini can also be used.

Try adding 3 oz (75 g) shrimp or cubed boneless chicken with pasta.

Make Ahead
This soup is best prepared just before serving so the pasta and vegetables do not get overcooked and lose their color.

1. In a large nonstick saucepan, heat oil over medium-high heat; add ginger, garlic, bok choy, green onions and 1/3 cup (75 mL) stock. Sauté, covered, for approximately 5 minutes.

2. Add 6 cups (1.5 L) stock; bring to boil and add soya sauce, vermicelli, snow peas, red peppers and tofu. Reduce heat to medium and cook for 3 minutes or until pasta is cooked.

Beef and bean couscous minestrone

Serves 8

Tip
Replace zucchini with broccoli or cauliflower for a change.

If bok choy or napa is unavailable, substitute romaine lettuce.

Couscous can be replaced with small shell pasta.

Make Ahead
Prepare soup up to a day in advance, but wait until reheating to add couscous, zucchini, green beans and bok choy. Add extra stock if too thick.

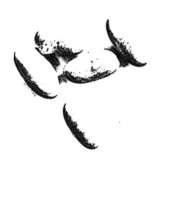

2 tsp	vegetable oil	10 mL
2 tsp	minced garlic	10 mL
1 cup	chopped onions	250 mL
1 cup	chopped carrots	250 mL
8 oz	diced round beef	250 g
5 cups	beef or chicken stock	1.25 L
1 cup	canned white kidney beans, drained	250 mL
1	can (19 oz [540 mL]) whole tomatoes	1
2	bay leaves	2
1 1/2 tsp	dried basil	7 mL
1/2 tsp	dried oregano	2 mL
1 cup	chopped zucchini	250 mL
1 cup	green beans	250 mL
1/4 cup	couscous	50 mL
2 cups	sliced bok choy or napa cabbage	500 mL
	Grated Parmesan cheese (optional)	

1. In a large saucepan sprayed with vegetable spray, heat oil over medium heat. Add garlic, onions and carrots; cook for 5 minutes or until onions and carrots are softened. Add beef and cook, stirring, for 3 to 5 minutes or until beef is no longer pink. Add stock, beans, tomatoes, bay leaves, basil and oregano; bring to a boil. Cover, reduce heat to low and simmer for 40 minutes or until carrots and beef are tender, stirring occasionally while crushing the tomatoes with back of a spoon.

2. Stir in zucchini, green beans and couscous. Cook, covered, for 10 minutes or until vegetables are tender. Stir in bok choy or cabbage; cook, covered, for 2 minutes or until wilted. Serve sprinkled with Parmesan cheese.

Moroccan spiced lentil soup

Serves 6

Most Mediterranean countries have their own version of this satisfying soup — a wonderful concoction of legumes, herbs and spices. Here's how it's made in North Africa. Serve with focaccia or pita bread and follow it with a lighter main course.

Make Ahead

Soup can be refrigerated, covered, for up to 3 days. Reheat over medium heat until piping hot, adding a little extra stock if soup has become too thick.

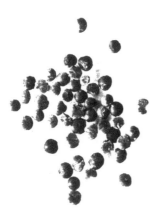

1 tbsp	olive oil	15 mL
2	onions, chopped	2
1	clove garlic, minced	1
1 tsp	ground ginger	5 mL
1 tsp	paprika	5 mL
1 tsp	turmeric	5 mL
1/4 tsp	cayenne pepper	1 mL
1 cup	red lentils, rinsed and drained	250 mL
4 cups	beef or chicken stock	1 L
1	can (28 oz [796 mL]) diced tomatoes	1
1	can (19 oz [540 mL]) chickpeas, rinsed and drained	1
1/3 cup	chopped fresh coriander	75 mL
1/4 tsp	salt	1 mL
1/4 tsp	black pepper	1 mL

1. In a large saucepan or Dutch oven, heat oil over medium-high heat. Add onions and garlic; cook, stirring, for 3 to 5 minutes or until onions are soft but not brown. Add ginger, paprika, turmeric and cayenne; cook, stirring, for about 1 minute. Add lentils; stir to coat with onion-and-spice mixture.

2. Add stock and tomatoes. Bring to a boil over high heat, stirring occasionally. Reduce heat to medium-low; simmer, covered, for 30 to 40 minutes or until lentils are very soft and have started to break up.

3. Stir in chickpeas, coriander, salt and pepper; simmer, uncovered, for 10 minutes to allow flavors to blend. If desired, season to taste with additional salt and pepper. Ladle into warm soup bowls. Serve at once.

Quick chickpea and pasta soup

Serves 4

Soup's on! Your fridge may be bare, but chances are you'll have the basic ingredients in your pantry to make this sustaining main-course soup for a quick-fix dinner.

Tip
Other types of canned beans or lentils can be used instead of chickpeas.

Variation
Chickpea, Pasta and Spinach Soup
Increase stock to 6 cups (1.5 L). Stir in 4 cups (1 L) shredded fresh spinach or Swiss chard, along with chickpeas and pasta.

1 tbsp	olive oil	15 mL
1	medium onion, chopped	1
2	cloves garlic, finely chopped	2
1/2 tsp	dried basil or Italian herbs	2 mL
2 tbsp	tomato paste	25 mL
5 cups	chicken stock or vegetable stock (approximate)	1.25 L
3/4 cup	small pasta shapes such as shells	175 mL
1	can (19 oz [540 mL]) chickpeas, rinsed and drained	1
	Salt and pepper	
	Grated Parmesan cheese	

1. In a large saucepan, heat oil over medium heat. Add onion, garlic and basil; cook, stirring, for 2 minutes or until softened. Add tomato paste; cook, stirring, for 30 seconds.
2. Add stock; bring to a boil. Stir in pasta and chickpeas; cook, partially covered and stirring occasionally, for 8 to 10 minutes or until pasta is just tender. Season with salt and pepper to taste. Ladle soup into bowls and serve sprinkled with Parmesan cheese.

Filipino black bean soup with shrimp

Serves 4

This hearty soup is most authentic with bitter melon (also known as bitter gourd) — a favorite throughout China and South/Southeast Asia. It has a decidedly bitter but fresh taste that takes some getting used to, but becomes quite addictive. It's good for you, too! Bitter melon aids digestion, cools the body and has antitoxic properties. At present, bitter melon is only available at Asian grocers, but I believe we will soon see it more frequently in North American markets.

Filipinos often use the tender leaves from the shoots of bitter melon vines to finish the soup; the leaves are even more bitter than the melons, but have an intense herbal flavor.

Another wonderful finishing touch for this soup is tender pea shoots, a fancy Asian vegetable that is also gaining a foothold in North American markets and is available during spring and autumn at Chinese grocers.

1 cup	black turtle beans	250 mL
4 tsp	dried shrimp	20 mL
1 tbsp	olive oil *or* vegetable oil	15 mL
3 oz	ground pork	75 g
1	small onion, chopped	1
2 tbsp	chopped celery	25 mL
1 tbsp	minced ginger root	15 mL
2 tsp	minced garlic	10 mL
1	bay leaf	1
1/4 tsp	black pepper	1 mL
2 tbsp	fish sauce or 2 tsp (10 mL) salt	25 mL
	Salt to taste	
1/4 cup	chopped red *or* green bell peppers	50 mL
Half	bitter melon (optional), seeded and cut into thin slices	Half
8 oz	shrimp, peeled and deveined	250 g
2 oz	fresh bitter melon leaves or pea shoots (optional)	50 g

1. In a bowl cover black beans with water and soak overnight. (Or use boiling water and let soak, covered, for 1 hour.) Drain; put beans in a large saucepan. Add 6 cups (1.5 L) water and bring to a boil. Reduce heat and simmer for 2 hours or until soft. Transfer two-thirds of the bean mixture to a food processor; purée and mix back with whole beans.

2. In a small bowl, cover dried shrimp with water; soak for 10 minutes. Drain; pound or chop shrimp to a fine powder.

3. In a heavy-bottomed pot, heat oil over medium heat. Add pork and fry until slightly browned. Stir in onion; cook 1 minute. Stir in celery, ginger, garlic, bay leaf, black pepper and dried shrimp; cook until fragrant. Add fish sauce and cook for 10 seconds. Add bean mixture and enough water for a thick soup consistency. Reduce heat to medium-low; cover and simmer for 10 minutes. Season to taste with salt.

4. Add chopped peppers and, if using, bitter melon; cook for 2 minutes or until vegetables are just tender. Add shrimp and simmer until cooked through. Add bitter melon leaves or pea shoots, if available, and simmer until they are just wilted.

Serves 8

The national dish of Greece, this economical, calorie-friendly, fuss-free, instantly likeable soup is chock full of flavor and nutrition. Its only drawback is that it requires hours and hours — almost days — to be ready. Normally I soak the beans overnight, and cook the soup the next day. I then refrigerate it (its flavor improves with time) and then reheat and serve it on the third day. It's worth the wait.

This soup is meant to be fairly thick; if too thick, add 1 to 2 cups (250 to 500 mL) water, stir and bring back to boil.

This recipe can be easily halved; but leftovers freeze well and can be reheated with minimal loss of flavor.

Fassolada
Greek bean soup

2 1/2 cups	dried white kidney beans	625 mL
1 tbsp	baking soda	15 mL
12 cups	water	3 L
1	onion, diced	1
1	large carrot, diced	1
1/2 cup	chopped fresh celery leaves, packed down (or 2 celery stalks, finely chopped)	125 mL
2 tbsp	tomato paste	25 mL
1 tsp	lemon juice	5 mL
1	medium tomato, blanched, skinned and chopped	1
1 tsp	dried rosemary, basil or oregano	5 mL
1 tsp	salt	5 mL
1/2 tsp	black pepper	2 mL
1/4 cup	chopped fresh parsley, packed down	50 mL
1/4 cup	olive oil	50 mL
	Extra virgin olive oil, olive bits, diced red onion, and crumbled feta cheese as accompaniments	

1. In a large bowl, cover beans with plenty of warm water. Add baking soda and mix well. (The water will foam and remove some of the gas from the beans.) Let soak for at least 3 hours, preferably overnight, unrefrigerated.

2. Drain beans and transfer to a soup pot. Add plenty of water and bring to a boil. Reduce heat to medium-low and simmer for 30 minutes, occasionally skimming any foam that rises to the top.

3. Drain beans; rinse and drain again. Scrub pot, cleaning off foam stuck to the sides. Return the beans to the pot; add the 12 cups (3 L) water and place over high heat. Add onion, carrot, celery, tomato paste, lemon juice and tomato. Bring to a boil, stirring; reduce heat to medium-low. Cook for 1 1/2 hours at a rolling boil, stirring very occasionally until the beans and vegetables are very tender.

4. Add rosemary, salt, pepper, parsley and olive oil. Cook for another 5 minutes, stirring occasionally, and take off heat. Cover soup and let rest for 5 to 10 minutes. If desired, season to taste with additional salt and pepper. Serve with any or all of suggested garnishes.

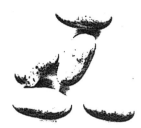

We recommend that you make the effort to find Madras curry powder for this recipe. (Look for it in Asian markets.) Rusty in color and usually containing bay leaves, it is fuller and more complex than regular curry powder, which contains more turmeric and tends to be bitter.

Curry-fried tofu soup with vegetables and udon noodles

Bouquet Garni

3	slices ginger root	3
1	clove garlic	1
1	stalk lemon grass, smashed and sliced *or* 1 tbsp (15 mL) lemon zest	1
2	star anise	2
2	thumb-sized pieces of dried tangerine peel, rinsed *or* 2 tsp (10 mL) orange zest	2

Soup

6 cups	vegetable or chicken stock	1.5 L
1	package (1 lb [500 g]) medium-firm tofu	1
2 tbsp	Madras curry powder	25 mL
1/4 tsp	salt	1 mL
4	packages (7 oz [200 g]) udon noodles *or* 1 lb (500 g) fresh spaghetti	4
2 cups	bean sprouts	500 mL
2 tbsp	vegetable oil	25 mL
1 cup	carrots, cut into matchsticks	250 mL
2 cups	broccoli florets	500 mL
1/2 tsp	salt	2 mL
4	sprigs cilantro	4

1. Wrap ingredients for bouquet garni in a piece of cheesecloth and tie securely with kitchen twine.

2. In a large saucepan or stock pot over high heat, bring bouquet garni and stock to a boil. Lower heat to medium and cook for 3 minutes. Cover and allow to steep for 15 minutes. Remove bouquet garni.

3. Cut tofu into 2-inch (5 cm) squares, about 1/2 inch (1 cm) thick. Pat dry with paper towels. In a mixing bowl, combine curry powder and salt; dredge tofu in mixture until lightly but evenly coated.

4. In a large pot of boiling salted water, cook noodles until *al dente*, about 2 minutes. Drain and divide between 4 serving bowls. Top with equally divided portions of bean sprouts.

5. In a nonstick wok or skillet, heat oil over medium-high heat for 30 seconds. Add tofu and fry until golden brown and slightly crisp on the outside, about 1 minute per side.

6. Meanwhile, bring broth to a boil. Add carrots and broccoli and cook for 3 minutes or until vegetables are just tender. Season with salt. Pour boiling broth and vegetables over noodle mixture. Top with tofu. Garnish with cilantro and serve immediately.

Serves 4 to 6

Mixed vegetable herb broth with soft tofu

The Asian flavor of miso, combined with traditional western herbs, enhances this savory vegetable soup.

1 tbsp	butter	15 mL
1/2 cup	diced onions	125 mL
1 cup	diced carrots	250 mL
5 cups	chicken stock *or* vegetable stock	1.25 L
3 tbsp	white or red miso paste	45 mL
1 cup	frozen peas	250 mL
1 cup	frozen corn kernels	250 mL
1 lb	soft tofu, cut into 1/2-inch (1 cm) cubes	500 g
2 tbsp	chopped basil	25 mL
2 tbsp	chopped parsley, preferably flat-leaf Italian variety	25 mL
1 tbsp	chopped chives	15 mL
	Seasoned salt and freshly ground black pepper to taste	

1. In a large saucepan or soup pot, melt butter over medium heat. Add onions and carrots; sauté for 1 minute. Add stock and miso and bring to a boil. Add peas and corn; cook for 2 minutes. Skim off any impurities that float to the top.

2. Gently stir tofu, basil, parsley and chives into the soup and return to a boil. Season to taste with seasoned salt and pepper. Remove from heat and serve immediately.

Spicy black bean gazpacho

Serves 6

A generous bowlful of this nourishing soup makes an ideal lunch or light supper. Just add some pita bread or whole grain crackers.

Tip
Tabasco is my preferred brand of hot pepper sauce, especially for tomato-based dishes.

Cold soups taste best when refrigerated overnight, giving the flavors a chance to blend. Always check the seasoning of a cold soup, however. Often you will need to add extra salt, pepper or hot pepper sauce.

1	red bell pepper, coarsely chopped	1
3	green onions, coarsely chopped	3
3	ripe tomatoes, coarsely chopped	3
1	large clove garlic, minced	1
1	can (19 oz [540 mL]) black beans, rinsed and drained	1
1	can (19 oz [540 mL]) tomato juice	1
2 tbsp	balsamic vinegar	25 mL
1 tbsp	red wine vinegar	15 mL
	Salt and pepper	
1/2 to 1 tsp	hot pepper sauce	2 to 5 mL
1/3 cup	chopped fresh coriander or parsley	75 mL
	Light sour cream *or* plain yogurt	

1. In a food processor, finely chop red pepper and green onions, using on-off turns; transfer to a large bowl. Add tomatoes to food processor; finely chop, using on-off turns. Add to pepper-onion mixture along with black beans and tomato juice. Add balsamic and red wine vinegars; season with salt, pepper and hot pepper sauce to taste. Cover and refrigerate for 4 hours, preferably overnight.

2. Add about 1/3 cup (75 mL) cold water to thin soup, if desired. Adjust seasoning with vinegars, salt, pepper and hot pepper sauce. Ladle into chilled bowls; sprinkle with coriander and top with a spoonful of sour cream.

Serves 4 to 6

Pumpkin and white bean soup

2 tsp	vegetable oil	10 mL
2 tsp	minced garlic	10 mL
1 cup	chopped onions	250 mL
1/2 cup	chopped carrots	125 mL
1/2 cup	chopped celery	125 mL
3 1/2 cups	vegetable stock	875 mL
1	can (14 oz [398 mL]) pumpkin (not pie filling)	1
1	can (19 oz [540 mL]) white kidney beans, rinsed and drained	1
1	bay leaf	1
1 tsp	ground ginger	5 mL
1/4 cup	maple syrup	50 mL

1. In a nonstick saucepan sprayed with vegetable spray, heat oil over medium-high heat. Add garlic, onions, carrots and celery; cook 4 minutes or until onions and celery are softened.

2. Stir in stock, pumpkin, beans, bay leaf and ginger. Bring to a boil; reduce heat and cook, covered, for 15 to 20 minutes or until vegetables are tender. Stir in maple syrup. Serve immediately.

Tip

In season, use fresh pumpkin. Bake approximately 1 hour at 375° F (190° C) or until tender.

If white kidney beans are unavailable, try small navy beans or chickpeas.

Maple syrup adds a subtle sweetness, unlike sugar.

This soup is a good source of fiber.

Make Ahead

Prepare up to 2 days in advance. Add more stock if too thick.

Freeze for up to 4 weeks.

Red bean and Ukrainian sausage soup

Serves 8

Ukrainian settlers came to the Canadian prairies as early as 1901, emigrating from Russia, Austria, Poland and other parts of Eastern Europe. Because they did not speak English, many worked as farm hands for more prosperous farmers; but soon they were cultivating their own land, with big gardens and mixed farms with cows and poultry. Their smoky garlic ham sausage is still available from Ukrainian butcher shops sprinkled throughout Western towns and cities — it's perfect for this hearty soup.

Use canned kidney beans, rinsed and drained or start with 2 cups (500 mL) dried kidney beans.

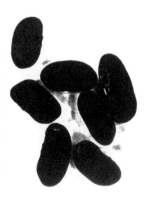

1	tomato, chopped	1
1	large onion, chopped	1
2	jalapeño peppers, seeded and chopped	2
6 oz	Ukranian sausage (kielbasa)	175 g
1 tbsp	chili powder	15 mL
1 tbsp	freshly ground black pepper	15 mL
1	bay leaf	1
2 tsp	red wine vinegar	10 mL
1	can (14 oz [398 mL]) whole stewed tomatoes, broken up	1
6 cups	beef stock	1.5 L
1/2 cup	ketchup *or* plain tomato sauce	125 mL
5 cups	cooked kidney beans	1.25 L
	Salt, granulated sugar and hot sauce to taste	

1. In a saucepan combine tomato, onion, jalapeño peppers, sausage, chili powder, pepper and bay leaf; cook over medium-high heat, covered and stirring occasionally, for 8 minutes or until tomatoes and onion have softened. Stir in vinegar. Add the stewed tomatoes, stock and ketchup and bring to a boil. Reduce heat to low and simmer, uncovered, for 1 hour.

2. Stir in beans and bring to a boil. Reduce heat and simmer for 10 minutes. Season to taste with salt, sugar and hot sauce.

Cabbage, bean and bacon chowder

Serves 6

The Great Northern bean is large and white, and is the North American version of the haricot bean or Italian cannellini bean. Substitute white kidney beans if Great Northern beans are unavailable.

2 tbsp	canola oil	25 mL
8 oz	lean Canadian back bacon, chopped	250 g
1	large onion, chopped	1
2	cloves garlic, minced	2
1	jalapeño pepper, seeded and chopped	1
2	carrots, chopped	2
1	potato, chopped	1
1	small white turnip, chopped	1
8 cups	beef stock	2 L
1 lb	green cabbage, finely shredded	500 g
1	can (19 oz [540 mL]) Great Northern beans, rinsed and drained	1
	Salt and pepper to taste	

1. In a large saucepan, heat oil over medium-high heat. Add back bacon, onion, garlic and jalapeño pepper; cook 4 minutes or until softened.
2. Stir in the carrots, potato, turnip and stock; bring to a boil. Reduce heat to medium-low and cook, covered, for 15 to 25 minutes or until vegetables are tender.
3. Stir in cabbage and cook for 15 minutes or until cabbage is tender. Stir in beans and heat through. Season to taste with salt and pepper.

Black bean and sausage gumbo

Serves 8 to 10

This hearty soup is really almost a stew. Serve it as a main course with cornbread and beer or ladle it over hot cooked rice in deep soup plates.

Use canned black beans, rinsed and drained, or start with 2 cups (500 mL) dried black beans.

1/2 cup	canola oil	125 mL
1/2 cup	all-purpose flour	125 mL
4	onions, chopped	4
4	stalks celery, chopped	4
1	red bell pepper, chopped	1
6	cloves garlic, pressed	6
8 cups	chicken stock	2 L
5 cups	cooked black beans	1.25 L
1/4 cup	Worcestershire sauce	50 mL
2 lbs	spicy Italian sausages, cooked and sliced	1 kg
1/2 tsp	chopped fresh thyme	2 mL
	Salt and pepper to taste	
1/2 cup	minced fresh parsley	125 mL
1/2 cup	chopped green onions	125 mL
1/2 cup	seeded and chopped tomatoes	125 mL
	Cornbread or hot cooked rice as accompaniment	

1. In a stock pot, cook oil and flour over medium heat, stirring constantly, for 10 minutes or until you have a brown roux the color of peanut butter. Be careful, this gets very hot and burns easily.

2. Stir in onions, celery, red pepper and garlic; cook, covered and stirring occasionally, for 8 minutes or until vegetables are tender. Stir in stock, beans, Worcestershire sauce, sausage and thyme; bring to a boil. Reduce heat to medium-low and cook, covered, for 30 minutes. Season to taste with salt and pepper. Stir in parsley and green onions. Place a mound of hot cooked rice in each serving bowl and spoon gumbo over top. Serve garnished with tomatoes.

Zuppa di lenticchie
Lentil soup with rice

Serves 6

If you can find them, use the small brown Italian lentils from Umbria or the dark green puy lentils – they don't break up during cooking, and they will nicely absorb any aromatics cooked with them, yet retain their attractive shape. Health food markets are good sources for a wide range of quality pulses, including organic varieties.

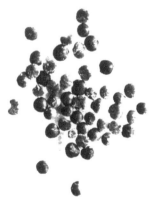

1 tbsp	butter	15 mL
1 tbsp	olive oil	15 mL
2	cloves garlic, finely chopped	2
1	small onion, finely chopped	1
1	stalk celery, finely chopped	1
1	small carrot, finely chopped	1
4 oz	pancetta, finely chopped	125 g
2 tbsp	finely chopped fresh marjoram	25 mL
1 1/2 cups	lentils, rinsed and drained	375 mL
1 1/2 cups	canned plum tomatoes with juices, finely chopped	375 mL
6 cups	beef stock	1.5 L
1/2 cup	short-grained Italian Arborio rice	125 mL
	Salt and freshly ground black pepper to taste	
1/2 cup	grated Parmigiano-Reggiano	125 mL
2 tbsp	chopped celery leaves	25 mL

1. In a saucepan with a lid, melt butter with olive oil over medium heat. Add garlic, onion, celery, carrot, pancetta and marjoram; sauté for 5 minutes or until vegetables have softened.

2. Stir in lentils and tomatoes; cook for 3 minutes. Add beef stock and bring to a boil. Reduce heat to low and cook, covered, for 30 minutes or until lentils are almost tender.

3. Stir in rice, replace cover and simmer, stirring occasionally, for another 20 minutes or until rice and lentils are tender. Season to taste with salt and pepper.

4. Serve sprinkled with Parmigiano-Reggiano and celery leaves.

Serves 6 to 8

Pasta e ceci
Pappardelle and chickpea soup

Pappardelle are long, ribbon-like strips of pasta, about 3/4 inch (2 cm) in width. They are often used with rich, creamy sauces, with porcini and, famously, with rabbit. This ancient version pairs the pasta with chickpeas as they do in Apulia where, just before serving, they often fry a little additional dried pasta at the very last minute to add another dimension of texture to the soup.

It's worth taking the time to use dried chickpeas and soak them overnight. Canned chickpeas are often over-cooked.

The rosemary is not traditional but works well with the chickpeas.

If using smaller canned plum tomatoes, add 2 to 3 more.

2 cups	dried chickpeas, soaked over-night in cold water to cover	500 mL
1	bay leaf	1
3 cups	vegetable stock *or* chicken stock	750 mL
1/4 cup	olive oil	50 mL
1	onion, chopped	1
3	cloves garlic, finely chopped	3
1	whole branch rosemary	1
3	large ripe plum tomatoes, peeled, seeded and chopped	3
	Salt and freshly ground black pepper to taste	
8 oz	pappardelle (or tagliatelle or fettuccine)	250 g
1/2 cup	chopped flat-leaf parsley	125 mL

1. In a large saucepan, combine drained chickpeas and bay leaf. Add cold water to cover by 2 inches (5 cm); bring to a boil. Reduce heat to simmer and cook for 1 hour or until chickpeas are tender. Drain, reserving cooking liquid. Wipe saucepan clean and return cooking liquid to saucepan. Add stock; bring to a boil and reduce heat to low.

2. In another large saucepan, heat olive oil over medium heat. Add onion, garlic and rosemary; cook for 5 minutes or until vegetables are softened. Stir in tomatoes; cook 5 minutes longer. Stir in stock mixture and chickpeas. Season to taste with salt and pepper. Bring to a boil; stir in pasta, reduce heat to simmer and cook, stirring occasionally, for 10 minutes or until pasta is tender. Remove rosemary. Serve sprinkled with parsley.

Serves 4 to 6

Zuppa di fagioli con biete
White bean soup with Swiss chard

This may be the best bean soup ever. The cooking time will depend on the freshness of the soaked beans. Health food stores are a good source for high-quality organic beans and pulses. Don't add salt to the beans' cooking water; this toughens them and encourages them to split open.

2 cups	dried cannellini beans (white kidney beans) or navy beans, soaked overnight in water to cover	500 mL
1 tbsp	olive oil	15 mL
8 oz	mushrooms, finely chopped (about 3 cups [750 mL])	250 g
3	cloves garlic, minced	3
1	onion, chopped	1
1/2 tsp	freshly grated nutmeg	2 mL
6 cups	chicken stock	1.5 L
1 lb	Swiss chard, washed, stemmed and chopped (about 6 cups [1.5 L])	500 g
	Salt and freshly ground black pepper to taste	
3 cups	ricotta cheese	750 mL
8	slices rustic country-style bread	8
3/4 cup	grated Pecorino Romano	175 mL
1/4 cup	chopped flat-leaf parsley	50 mL

1. Drain beans and place in a large saucepan. Add water to cover by 2 inches (5 cm); bring to a boil. Reduce heat to simmer and cook for 1 1/2 hours or until beans are tender, skimming any foam that rises to the surface. Drain beans, discarding cooking liquid.

2. Wipe saucepan clean. Heat olive oil in saucepan over medium heat. Add mushrooms, garlic, onion and nutmeg; cook, stirring often, for 5 minutes or until vegetables are softened. Stir in cooked beans and chicken stock; bring to a boil. Reduce heat to medium-low and cook for 20 minutes. Stir in Swiss chard; cook for 2 minutes or until wilted. Season to taste with salt and pepper.

3. Preheat broiler. Spread ricotta cheese on bread slices. Top with Pecorino Romano. Broil for 2 minutes or until cheese is golden.

4. Ladle soup into soup plates. Place a piece of cheese toast in the center of each serving. Sprinkle with parsley. Serve with extra toasts on the side.

Savory red lentil soup

Lentils were once considered "poor man's food" but that poor person could have done worse. This prehistoric legume is extremely high in protein and is also rich in minerals. Red lentils are often used in Indian dal, croquettes and curries. Here they make a hearty soup delicious. Organically grown lentils, and many other organic legumes, are widely available.

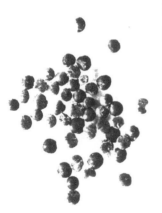

1/4 cup	olive oil	50 mL
1	large onion, chopped	1
1	large carrot, sliced	1
2	cloves garlic, chopped	2
1 tsp	dried thyme	5 mL
1 tbsp	dried marjoram	15 mL
1/4 tsp	curry powder (optional)	1 mL
5 cups	vegetable stock	1.25 L
1 1/2 cups	red lentils	375 mL
1/4 cup	chopped parsley	50 mL
3	medium tomatoes, chopped	3
	Salt and pepper to taste	
1/4 cup	red wine	50 mL
1 cup	grated sharp Cheddar cheese (optional)	250 mL

1. In a large heavy-bottomed pot with a lid, heat oil over medium heat. Add onion, carrot, garlic, thyme, marjoram and, if using, curry; sauté for 6 minutes or until onion is transparent.

2. Add vegetable stock, red lentils, parsley and tomatoes. Season to taste with salt and pepper. Cover and simmer for 1 hour. (Add more stock, if necessary, to achieve desired consistency.)

3. Add red wine just before serving. Garnish with grated sharp Cheddar cheese, if desired.

Pasta fagioli Capra
Bean and pasta soup Capra

Serves 6

A long-time favorite soup, pasta fagioli combines beans, pasta and vegetables to make a delicious meal-in-a-bowl. Italian-born Toronto chef Massimo Capra, of Mistura Restaurant, makes a version that uses different types of beans. The actual combination of beans can be varied to suit your taste and may either be canned, dried, fresh or frozen. If using canned beans, rinse and drain well.

One day I was wondering what to do with leftovers of this soup and some soft polenta. So I shaped the polenta into small patties, fried them in a little butter, placed them in the bottom of a shallow soup plate and poured the hot soup over to cover slightly. Ambrosial!

3 tbsp	extra virgin olive oil	45 mL
1	stalk celery, finely chopped	1
1	small onion, finely chopped	1
1	small carrot, finely chopped	1
6	cloves garlic, finely chopped	6
1	sprig thyme, leaves only, finely chopped	1
2	bay leaves	2
1 cup	chopped plum tomatoes, canned or fresh	250 mL
1/4 cup	cooked romano beans	50 mL
1/4 cup	cooked black-eyed peas	50 mL
1/4 cup	cooked cannellini beans (white kidney beans) or navy beans	50 mL
1/4 cup	cooked large lima beans	50 mL
1/4 cup	cooked chickpeas	50 mL
6 cups	vegetable stock	1.5 L
	Salt and freshly ground black pepper	
	Freshly grated nutmeg	
1 cup	maccheroni (the straight, short variety) or ditalini or tubetti	250 mL
1/2 cup	cooked peeled fava beans	125 mL
1/4 cup	roughly chopped flat-leaf parsley	50 mL
	Olive oil	
6	slices of rustic country-style bread brushed with olive oil and grilled or oven-toasted	6

1. In a large saucepan, heat olive oil over medium heat. Add celery, onion, carrot, garlic, thyme and bay leaves; cook for 5 minutes or until vegetables are softened. Stir in tomatoes; cook, stirring, for 3 minutes.

2. Stir in romano beans, black-eyed peas, kidney beans, lima beans and chickpeas. Add stock and bring to a boil. Reduce heat to simmer and cook for 15 minutes, skimming any foam that rises to the top. Season to taste with salt, pepper and nutmeg.

3. Stir in pasta and fava beans; return to a simmer and cook, stirring occasionally, for 10 minutes or just until pasta is tender.

4. Stir in parsley. Drizzle with olive oil and serve immediately with toasts.

Ribollita
Thick bean soup

Serves 6 to 8

Hearty bean soups are almost a way of life in Italy — especially in Tuscany, where the residents have long been known as *mangia fagioli* or "bean eaters." Sustaining, filling and satisfying, these soups (which also include minestrone or *pasta fagioli*) form the basis of the next day's supper. This is the inspiration for sturdy *ribollita*, which means "reboiled."

12-CUP (3 L) SOUP TUREEN OR CASSEROLE DISH

3 tbsp	olive oil	45 mL
3	cloves garlic, finely chopped	3
2	medium leeks, green part only, trimmed, washed and finely chopped	2
1	onion, finely chopped	1
1	carrot, finely chopped	1
1	stalk celery, finely chopped	1
2 tsp	finely chopped rosemary	10 mL
1	small dried chili pepper	1
1 1/4 cups	dried cannellini beans (white kidney beans) or navy beans, soaked overnight in water to cover	300 mL
	Salt and freshly ground black pepper to taste	
1/2 cup	extra virgin olive oil	125 mL
2	cloves garlic, crushed	2
2	whole sprigs thyme	2
8	slices oven-toasted or grilled bread, brushed with olive oil and rubbed with garlic	8
1 cup	grated Parmigiano-Reggiano	250 mL

1. In a large saucepan, heat olive oil over medium heat. Add garlic, leeks, onion, carrot, celery, rosemary and chili; cook, stirring frequently, for 10 minutes or until vegetables are softened and starting to brown. Stir in drained beans and 10 cups (2.5 L) water. Bring to a boil; reduce heat to simmer and cook 1 1/2 hours or until beans are tender, skimming any foam that rises to the surface.

2. With a slotted spoon, transfer half of the cooked beans and vegetables to a food processor or blender; purée. Return bean purée to saucepan; stir to blend. Season to taste with salt and pepper. Keep soup at a low simmer.

3. Preheat oven to 375° F (190° C). In a small skillet, heat olive oil over medium heat. Add garlic and thyme; cook for 2 minutes or until garlic is golden. Strain oil into a heatproof bowl; discard solids.

4. Put toasts in bottom of soup tureen or casserole dish; sprinkle with half of the cheese. Pour bean soup over toasts. Drizzle garlic-thyme oil over the surface. Sprinkle with remaining cheese. Bake, uncovered, for 30 minutes or until cheese is golden. Serve from tureen at the table.

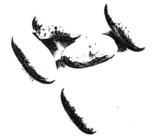

Lamb soup with red wine, romano beans and chèvre

Serves 10

This soup is really a meal in itself — and the smell of it simmering in the oven is mouthwatering. If you want to scale down this recipe, you can use a smaller cut of lamb, such as a center leg roast.

Unlike beef, where there are many cuts of meat, lamb offers a more limited selection. A leg of lamb, which comes from the rear leg of the animal, can be bought in a number of ways. The heavier the leg, the older and fattier the lamb. (Generally, to be called a lamb, the animal must be under 1 year old.) Look for pink meat with creamy white fat.

PREHEAT OVEN TO 375° F (190° C)

1	leg of lamb (about 5 to 6 lbs [2.5 to 3 kg])	1
	Salt and pepper	
2 tbsp	olive oil	25 mL
2 tbsp	butter	25 mL
2	onions, chopped	2
2	carrots, chopped	2
2	parsnips, chopped	2
1	fennel bulb, cored and chopped	1
2	cloves garlic, pressed	2
1/2 cup	red currant jelly	125 mL
1/2 cup	balsamic vinegar	125 mL
3 cups	red wine	750 mL
4 cups	water	1 L
1 lb	plum tomatoes, chopped	500 g
1 cup	Romano beans, soaked overnight and drained	250 mL
1	bay leaf	1
	Fresh thyme, to taste	
	Fresh tarragon, to taste	
	Freshly grated Parmesan cheese	
	Fresh chèvre (goat cheese), crumbled	
	Zest of 1 orange	

1. Season the lamb with salt and pepper. In a large, heavy ovenproof casserole dish with a lid, heat olive oil and butter over medium-high heat until bubbling. Add lamb and sear on all sides until browned. Place casserole in preheated oven and roast for 45 minutes. Remove from oven and, with a slotted spoon, transfer lamb to a bowl.

2. To the casserole dish, add onions, carrots, parsnips and fennel; cook over medium heat until browned. Add pressed garlic and cook for 2 minutes or until slightly browned.

3. Stir in red currant jelly, balsamic vinegar, wine, water, tomatoes and Romano beans. Add the lamb along with the bay leaf, thyme and tarragon. Cover and simmer in the oven for another hour.

4. Remove casserole from oven. Cut lamb into pieces and return to stock. Adjust seasoning and serve in warm bowls, garnished with Parmesan, crumbled chèvre and orange zest.

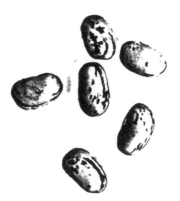

Mexican corn, bean and pasta soup

Serves 6 to 8

Tip
Chickpeas or other beans can replace kidney beans.

Any small shell pasta can be used.

Make Ahead
Prepare soup up to a day ahead, but do not add pasta until 10 minutes before serving.

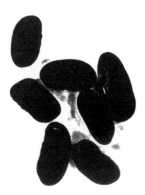

2 tsp	vegetable oil	10 mL
2 tsp	crushed garlic	10 mL
1 cup	chopped onions	250 mL
1 1/2 cups	chopped green bell peppers	375 mL
1	can (28 oz [796 mL]) crushed tomatoes	1
2 1/2 cups	chicken stock	625 mL
2 cups	canned red kidney beans, drained	500 mL
1 cup	corn niblets	250 mL
1 tbsp	chili powder	15 mL
1/4 tsp	cayenne pepper	1 mL
1/2 cup	macaroni	125 mL
Dollop	yogurt	Dollop
	Fresh coriander	

1. In a large nonstick saucepan, heat oil over medium-high heat; sauté garlic, onions and green peppers for 5 minutes or until soft.
2. Add tomatoes, stock, beans, corn niblets, chili powder and cayenne. Reduce heat to low and simmer, covered, for 20 minutes.
3. Add pasta and simmer for 10 to 12 minutes or until pasta is "al dente" (firm to the bite). Garnish with yogurt and fresh coriander.

Salads

Cajun potato and red lentil salad

Serves 4

Tip
Double the amounts for a summer picnic or barbecue.

If not accustomed to cayenne pepper, start with 1/4 tsp (1 mL) and gradually add more to taste.

Large sprouts such as broccoli or sunflower work well in this recipe, but you can use any type available.

Variations
Substitute: Green onions for scapes; Sour cream for yogurt; More or less cayenne pepper, to taste.

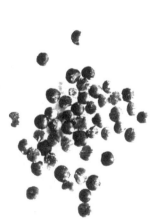

1/2 cup	red lentils, rinsed	125 mL
1 1/2 cups	water	375 mL
4	large potatoes, scrubbed and halved	4
1/3 cup	flaxseed oil	75 mL
3 tbsp	raspberry vinegar	45 mL
2 tbsp	sesame seeds	25 mL
2 tbsp	poppy seeds	25 mL
2 tbsp	flax seeds	25 mL
1/3 cup	plain yogurt	75 mL
1 tsp	cayenne powder	5 mL
	Salt and black pepper	
1/4 cup	chopped scapes	50 mL
3	hardboiled eggs, cut into wedges	3
1/4 cup	large sprouts (see Tip, at left)	50 mL

1. In a saucepan combine lentils with water. Bring to a boil; reduce heat and simmer gently for 20 minutes or until lentils are tender. Allow to cool in a colander.

2. Meanwhile, in a medium saucepan, cover potatoes with cold water. Bring to a boil, reduce heat and simmer for 20 to 25 minutes or until just tender. Drain and rinse with cold water. When cool enough to handle, cut into 1-inch (2.5 cm) pieces.

3. In a small bowl, whisk together oil, raspberry vinegar, sesame seeds, poppy seeds, flax seeds, yogurt and cayenne. Season to taste with salt and pepper.

4. In a large salad bowl, combine cooled lentils, potatoes and scapes. Gently stir in dressing. Garnish with egg wedges and sprouts.

POTATO AND CHICKPEA STEW WITH SPICY SAUSAGE (PAGE 80) ➤
OVERLEAF, LEFT: GREEK CHILI WITH BLACK OLIVES AND FETA CHEESE (PAGE 89)
OVERLEAF, RIGHT: SALMON OVER WHITE-AND-BLACK BEAN SALSA (PAGE 124)

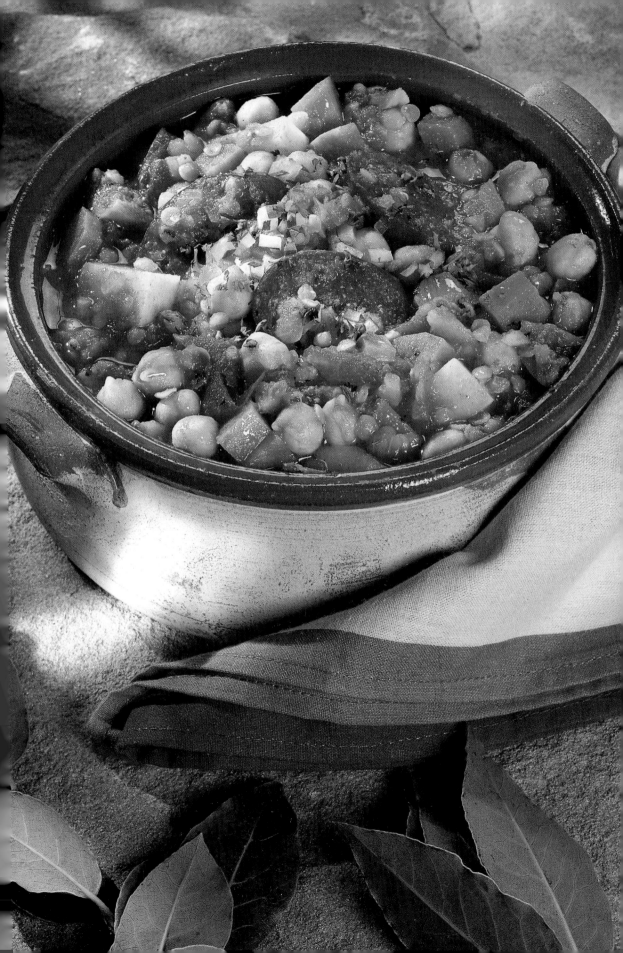

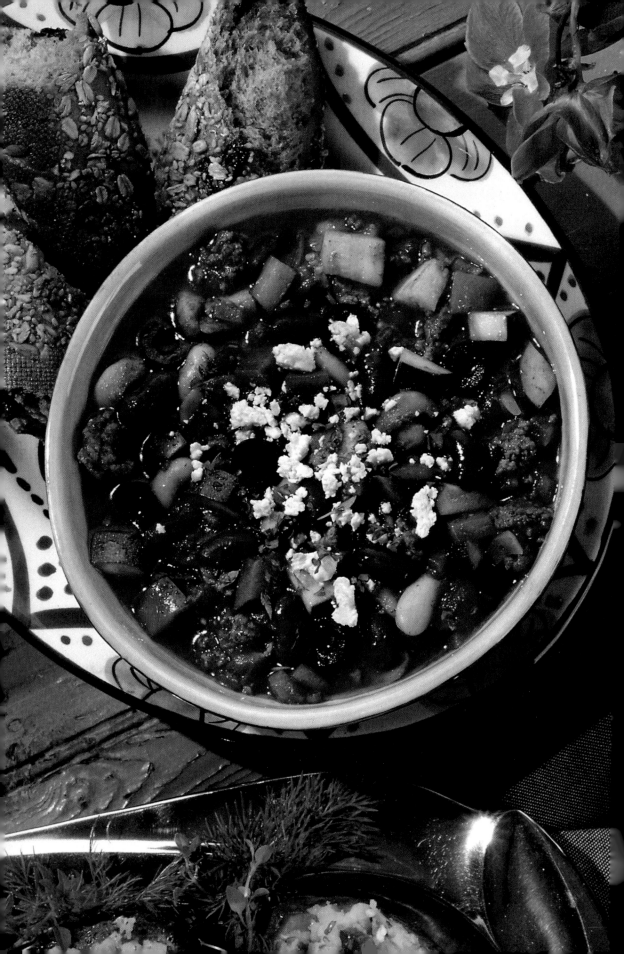

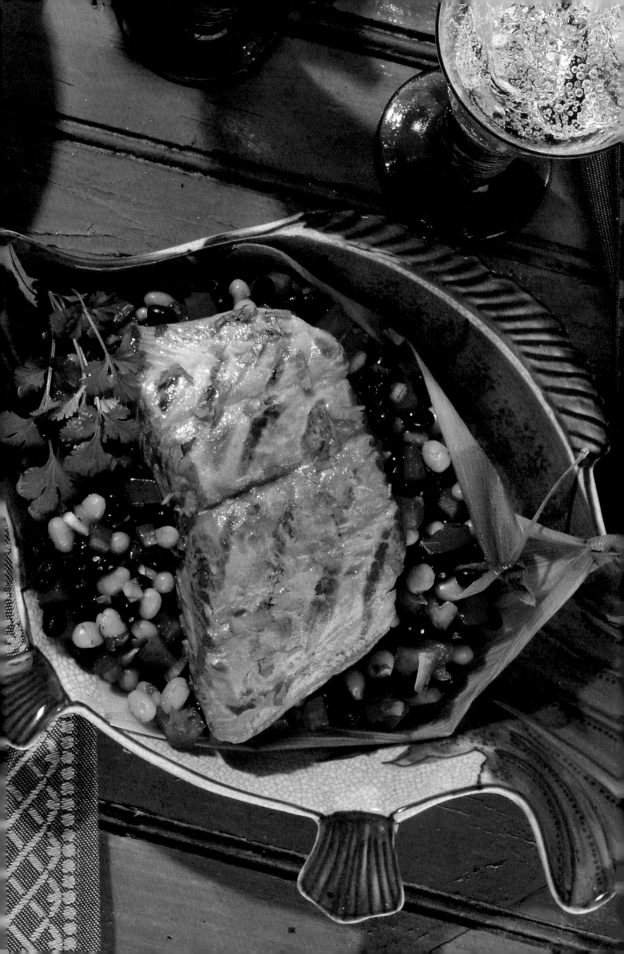

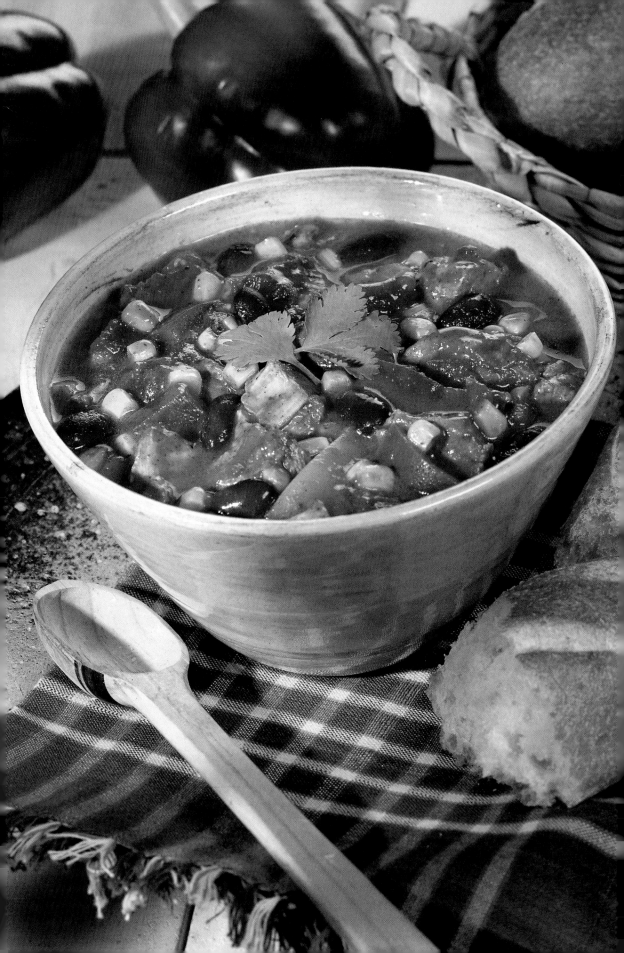

Italian bean pasta salad

Serves 6 to 8 as an appetizer

Tip
Use any combination of cooked beans. Try black beans or lima beans.

Make Ahead
Prepare salad and dressing early in the day. Toss up to 2 hours ahead.

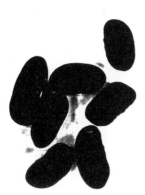

12 oz	medium shell pasta	375 g
2 1/2 cups	chopped tomatoes	625 mL
3/4 cup	diced green bell peppers	175 mL
3/4 cup	diced red onions	175 mL
2/3 cup	canned red kidney beans, drained	150 mL
2/3 cup	canned white kidney beans, drained	150 mL
2/3 cup	canned chickpeas, drained	150 mL
3 oz	feta cheese, crumbled	75 g

Dressing

1/4 cup	lemon juice	50 mL
3 tbsp	olive oil	45 mL
1 tbsp	red wine vinegar	15 mL
2 tsp	crushed garlic	10 mL
2 1/2 tsp	dried basil	12 mL
1 1/2 tsp	dried oregano	7 mL

1. Cook pasta in boiling water according to package instructions or until firm to the bite. Rinse with cold water. Drain and place in a serving bowl. Add tomatoes, green peppers, onions, red kidney beans, white kidney beans, chickpeas and feta cheese.

2. Make the dressing: In a small bowl, whisk together lemon juice, oil, vinegar, garlic, basil and oregano. Pour over pasta and toss.

≺ MAKE-AHEAD SOUTHWESTERN PORK STEW (PAGE 86)

Corn and three-bean salad

Serves 6 to 8

Tip
Use any combination of cooked beans.

For a sweeter salad, try balsamic vinegar.

Make ahead
Prepare salad and dressing separately up to a day ahead. Pour dressing over top just before serving.

8 oz	pasta wheels or small shell pasta	250 g
1 cup	canned black beans or chickpeas, drained	250 mL
3/4 cup	canned red kidney beans, drained	175 mL
3/4 cup	canned white kidney beans, drained	175 mL
3/4 cup	canned corn niblets, drained	175 mL
1 1/4 cups	diced red bell peppers	300 mL
3/4 cup	diced carrots	175 mL
1/2 cup	diced red onions	125 mL

Dressing

1/4 cup	lemon juice	50 mL
3 tbsp	vegetable oil	45 mL
3 tbsp	red wine or cider vinegar	45 mL
2 tsp	crushed garlic	10 mL
1/2 cup	chopped coriander or parsley	125 mL

1. Cook pasta in boiling water according to package instructions or until firm to the bite. Rinse with cold water. Drain and place in a serving bowl.
2. Add black beans, red kidney beans, white kidney beans, corn niblets, red peppers, carrots and onions.
3. Make the dressing: In a small bowl, combine lemon juice, oil, wine, garlic and coriander. Pour over dressing and toss.

Bean salad with mustard-dill dressing

Serves 6

Bean salad is another staple we've grown up with over the years. Originally this salad used canned string beans, but fresh beans give it a new lease on taste, as does the addition of fiber-packed chickpeas.

Tip
Instead of chickpeas, you can try canned mixed beans. This includes a combination of chickpeas, red and white kidney beans and black-eyed peas. It's available in super-markets.

Variation
French Salad Dressing
In a bowl, stir together 2 tbsp (25 mL) red wine vinegar and 1 1/2 tsp (7 mL) Dijon mustard. Add 1/3 cup (75 mL) olive oil (or use part vegetable oil), 1 minced clove garlic and 1 tsp (5 mL) dried fine herbs. Season with a pinch of granulated sugar, salt and pepper to taste. Store in covered jar in the refrigerator. Makes 1/2 cup (125 mL).

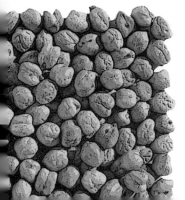

1 lb	green beans	500 g
1	can (19 oz [540 mL]) chickpeas, rinsed and drained	1
1/3 cup	chopped red onions	75 mL
2 tbsp	finely chopped fresh dill	25 mL
2 tbsp	olive oil	25 mL
2 tbsp	red wine vinegar	25 mL
1 tbsp	Dijon mustard	15 mL
1 tbsp	granulated sugar	15 mL
1/4 tsp	salt	1 mL
1/4 tsp	pepper	1 mL

1. Trim ends of beans; cut into 1-inch (2.5 cm) lengths. In a large pot of boiling salted water, cook beans for 3 to 5 minutes (count from time water returns to boil) or until tender-crisp. Drain; rinse under cold water to chill. Drain well.

2. In a serving bowl, combine green beans, chickpeas, onions and dill.

3. In a small bowl, whisk together oil, vinegar, mustard, sugar, salt and pepper until smooth. Pour over beans and toss well. Refrigerate until serving time.

Serves 4

Tortilla chips are a great snack food — but only if they're baked! The traditional deep-fried variety is much higher in fat and calories.

For a great snack, melt some light Cheddar cheese over tortillas. Kids love them!

Tex-Mex rotini salad

8 oz	rotini	250 g
1 1/2 cups	diced ripe plum tomatoes	375 mL
1 cup	canned red kidney beans, rinsed and drained	250 mL
1 cup	canned corn kernels, rinsed and drained	250 mL
1/2 cup	chopped fresh coriander	125 mL
1/2 cup	chopped green onions	125 mL

Dressing

1/3 cup	barbecue sauce	75 mL
2 1/2 tbsp	cider vinegar	35 mL
2 tsp	molasses	10 mL
1 tsp	minced jalapeño pepper (optional)	5 mL
1 oz	baked tortilla chips (about 12)	25 g

1. In a large pot of boiling water, cook rotini for 8 to 10 minutes or until tender but firm; drain. Rinse under cold running water; drain. In a serving bowl combine pasta, tomatoes, kidney beans, corn, coriander and green onions.
2. In a bowl combine barbecue sauce, cider vinegar, molasses and jalapeño pepper; whisk well. Pour dressing over salad; toss to coat well. Garnish with crumbled tortilla chips. Serve.

White bean salad with lemon-dill vinaigrette

Serves 6 to 8

Bean salads can be so disappointing. But this one is fresh-tasting and holds up well for several hours without refrigeration — perfect for a buffet table.

Kitchen Wisdom

Dill is one of the few fresh herbs that freeze well. Simply place in a plastic bag and freeze for up to 6 months. To use, just break off what you need from the frozen bunch. For best results, add to cooked dishes rather than salads.

Make Ahead

The bean salad can be refrigerated for up to 8 hours. Let stand at room temperature for 30 minutes before serving.

2	cans (each 19 oz [540 mL]) white kidney beans, rinsed and drained	2
2	small tomatoes, chopped	2
1/2 cup	finely chopped red onion	125 mL
1/4 cup	chopped fresh dill	50 mL
1/4 cup	olive oil	50 mL
2 tbsp	fresh lemon juice	25 mL
1 tbsp	liquid honey	15 mL
1/4 tsp	salt	1 mL
1/4 tsp	black pepper	1 mL

1. In a large serving bowl, combine beans, tomatoes, onion and 3 tbsp (45 mL) dill.

2. In a small bowl, whisk together olive oil, lemon juice, honey, salt and pepper. Add to beans; toss well. If desired, season to taste with additional salt and pepper. Serve garnished with remaining dill.

Rice, black bean and red pepper salad

Serves 6

Tip
This recipe can be prepared using all wild rice or all white rice.

Canned black beans can be difficult to find. Cook your own dry beans — 1/2 cup (125 mL) of dry beans yields approximately 1 1/2 cups (375 mL) cooked. Cook in simmering water for 1 hour or until beans are tender. Otherwise, any other canned beans can be used.

For best taste, allow to chill before serving.

Make Ahead
Prepare entire salad early in the day, keeping refrigerated. Stir well before serving.

2 cups	chicken stock *or* water	500 mL
1/2 cup	wild rice	125 mL
1/2 cup	white rice	125 mL
1 cup	chopped red bell peppers	250 mL
1 cup	chopped snow peas	250 mL
1 cup	canned black beans, drained	250 mL
1/2 cup	corn kernels	125 mL
1/3 cup	chopped red onions	75 mL
1/3 cup	chopped fresh coriander or parsley	75 mL
1	medium green onion, chopped	1

Dressing

3 tbsp	olive oil	45 mL
2 tbsp	lemon juice	25 mL
1 tbsp	red wine vinegar	15 mL
1 tsp	minced garlic	5 mL

1. In a saucepan bring stock or water to a boil; add wild rice and white rice. Cover, reduce heat to medium-low and simmer for 20 minutes or until rice is tender. Remove from heat and let stand for 5 minutes or until all liquid is absorbed. Rinse with cold water and put in a large serving bowl.

2. Add red peppers, snow peas, black beans, corn, red onions, coriander and green onion to rice; toss to combine.

3. In a small bowl, whisk together olive oil, lemon juice, red wine vinegar and garlic; pour over salad and toss well.

Tortilla bean salad with creamy salsa dressing

Serves 4

Tip
Southwestern all the way, this salad is low in fat — thanks to the light dressing.

Use a mild or hot salsa, whichever you prefer.

Vary beans and vegetables to your taste.

To prevent salad from wilting, do not pour dressing over until ready to serve.

Make Ahead
Prepare salad and dressing early in the day. Toss just before serving.

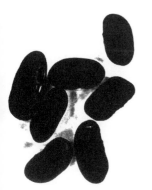

Salad

3 cups	romaine lettuce, washed, dried and torn into pieces	750 mL
1 cup	canned chickpeas, rinsed and drained	250 mL
1 cup	canned red kidney beans, rinsed and drained	250 mL
1 cup	shredded carrots	250 mL
1 cup	chopped red bell peppers	250 mL
3/4 cup	chopped red onions	175 mL
1/3 cup	chopped fresh coriander	75 mL

Dressing

3 tbsp	salsa	45 mL
3 tbsp	light sour cream	45 mL
2 tbsp	light mayonnaise	25 mL
1 tsp	minced garlic	5 mL
3/4 to 1 tsp	chili powder	4 to 5 mL
1 oz	tortilla chips, crushed (about 12)	25 g

1. In a large bowl, combine lettuce, chickpeas, kidney beans, carrots, red peppers, red onions and coriander.
2. Make the dressing: In a small bowl, whisk together salsa, sour cream, mayonnaise, garlic and chili powder.
3. Just before serving, pour dressing over salad. Toss to coat. Sprinkle with tortilla chips. Serve immediately.

Serves 4 to 6

Lentil and beet salad

Writer-producer, ex(traordi-nary) neighbor, and all-around fabulous person, Sharon Corder, created this earthy/swarthy salad for the dinner parties she and hubby Jack Blum seem to throw at will. It's surprisingly light, considering its weighty ingredients, and easy to make — save for the time it takes to boil those pesky beets (and cleaning up the blood-red stains that inevitably result).

If possible, prepare your own lentils instead of using the canned variety. Use 1 cup (250 mL) dry lentils to get 2 cups (500 mL) cooked.

1 lb	beets, unpeeled but well scrubbed	500 g
2 cups	cooked green lentils	500 mL
1/2 cup	finely diced red bell peppers	125 mL
1/4 cup	finely diced red onions	50 mL
1	stick celery, finely diced	1
1 tbsp	lemon zest	15 mL
1 tbsp	walnut oil	15 mL
1/2 tsp	ground cumin	2 mL
1/2 cup	chopped walnuts	125 mL
3 tbsp	lemon juice	45 mL
1 tbsp	red wine vinegar	15 mL
1 tsp	Worcestershire sauce	5 mL
3	cloves garlic, minced	3
Pinch	nutmeg	Pinch
3 tbsp	walnut oil	45 mL
	Salt and pepper to taste	
1	bunch beet greens	1
	Few sprigs fresh dill, chopped	

1. Place beets in a large saucepan and add enough water to cover by 1 1/2 inches (3 cm). Bring to a boil and cook beets for 50 to 60 minutes or until they can be pierced easily with a fork. If water evaporates to expose beets during cooking, replenish with more hot water. Drain the liquid and allow the beets to cool; peel, trim, and cut into 1/4-inch (0.5 cm) cubes.

2. Transfer the beets to a bowl. Add lentils, red peppers, red onions, celery and lemon zest. Mix thoroughly. The salad will have turned a dark red.

3. In a small frying pan, heat the walnut oil over medium-high heat for 30 seconds. Add ground cumin and stir for 30 seconds. Add chopped walnuts and stir-fry for 2 minutes or until starting to brown. Add to the salad, scraping off the cumin and oil from the pan; toss gently.

4. In a small bowl, whisk together lemon juice, vinegar, Worcestershire sauce, garlic and nutmeg; add walnut oil, whisking to emulsify. Pour over the salad and fold everything together. Season to taste with salt and pepper.

5. Steam or boil the beet greens for no more than 2 minutes; drain immediately and refresh in iced water. Trim the stalks and discard. Arrange the leaves around the rim of a serving plate.

6. Transfer salad to the center of the plate and garnish liberally with chopped dill. This salad can be served immediately or it can wait for up to 2 hours, covered and unrefrigerated.

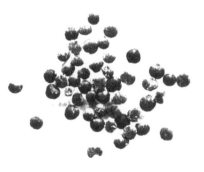

Serves 8

Black bean and rice salad

This colorful salad makes a great summer meal or portable potluck offering. It's also very Western with Tex-Mex overtones and earthy black beans.

1 cup	dried black beans, soaked overnight in water to cover	250 mL
1	onion, halved	1
2	cloves garlic, chopped	2
1	small carrot	1
1	sprig fresh parsley	1
1 cup	white rice	250 mL
1 tbsp	canola oil	15 mL
1 tsp	turmeric	5 mL
1/2 tsp	ground cumin	2 mL
1/2 tsp	salt	2 mL

Dressing

3 tbsp	olive oil	45 mL
3 tbsp	fresh lime juice	45 mL
1/2 tsp	ground cumin	2 mL
2	tomatoes, seeded and diced	2
1	small red onion, diced	1
1	red bell pepper, diced	1
1	jalapeño pepper, seeded and minced	1
1/4 cup	chopped cilantro	50 mL
	Cayenne pepper to taste	

1. In a saucepan combine drained beans with 8 cups (2 L) cold water, onion, garlic, carrot and parsley; bring to a boil. Reduce heat and simmer for 1 1/2 hours or until tender. Drain and cool. Discard onion, carrot and parsley.

2. Meanwhile, in a small saucepan combine 1 3/4 cups (425 mL) cold water, rice, oil, turmeric, cumin and salt; bring to a boil. Reduce heat to low and simmer, covered, for 30 minutes. Fluff rice and cool to room temperature.

3. Make the dressing: In a small bowl, whisk together olive oil, lime juice and cumin. Set aside.

4. In a large bowl, toss cooled beans and rice with tomatoes, red onion, red pepper, jalapeño, cilantro and dressing. Season to taste with cayenne pepper and, if desired, additional salt. Chill.

Serves 4 to 6

Baby fava bean and pecorino salad

In Italy, this salad is prepared in May when the fava (broad) beans are only just formed and still dozing in their lovely fuzz-lined pods. They are enjoyed uncooked, treated to the very best extra virgin olive oil and then paired with small cubes of young Pecorino. If you cannot find a young version of this sheep's milk cheese, substitute Emmental or even a mild Cheddar. The quantity of fresh beans may seem like a lot, but remember they are still in the pod, which adds to their weight. Use your very finest olive oil for this dish.

5 lbs	young fava beans (in pods)	2.5 kg
	Salt and freshly ground black pepper to taste	
1/4 cup	extra virgin olive oil	50 mL
12 oz	young Pecorino Romano, cut into neat 1/2-inch (1 cm) cubes	375 g
	Crusty bread	

1. Pod the beans and place in a medium-size bowl. Season with salt and pepper. Add olive oil gradually and toss to make sure all beans are well coated. (The beans should not be floating in oil.)

2. Add cubes of cheese and toss once or twice. Serve at once with crusty bread to mop up the oil.

Serves 8

Bean salads and macaroni salads are standard fare at western hoe-downs and prairie picnics. Here's a recipe that combines the best of both with a few new twists, a favorite of mine for summer barbecues and potluck dinners.

For convenience, use 1 can (14 oz [398 mL]) kidney beans and 1 can (14 oz [398 mL]) chickpeas, rinsed and drained.

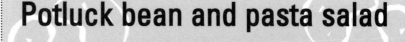

Potluck bean and pasta salad

Dressing

2 tbsp	red wine vinegar	25 mL
1 tbsp	fresh lemon juice	15 mL
1 tbsp	Dijon mustard	15 mL
2 tsp	Worcestershire sauce	10 mL
1 tsp	granulated sugar	5 mL
1/2 tsp	salt	2 mL
1/4 tsp	freshly ground black pepper	1 mL
2	cloves garlic	2
1/2 cup	extra virgin olive oil	125 mL
2 tbsp	minced fresh parsley	25 mL
1 tbsp	basil pesto or minced fresh basil	15 mL
3 cups	short pasta (small shells, rotini or radiatore)	750 mL
1 1/2 cups	cooked kidney beans	375 mL
1 1/2 cups	cooked chickpeas	375 mL
1 cup	diced yellow peppers	250 mL
1/2 cup	sliced black olives	125 mL
3	large plum tomatoes, seeded and chopped	3
Half	red onion, diced	Half
	Salt and pepper to taste	

1. Make the dressing: In a small glass measuring cup, whisk together vinegar, lemon juice, mustard, Worcestershire sauce, sugar, salt and pepper; set aside. In a food processor, chop garlic. Add vinegar mixture and process until well mixed. With machine running, slowly pour olive oil, parsley and pesto through feed tube. Set aside.

2. In a large pot of boiling, salted water, cook pasta for 8 to 10 minutes or until al dente; drain. Rinse under cold running water; drain again, shaking well to remove any excess water.

3. In a large bowl, toss together pasta, kidney beans, chickpeas and dressing. Add yellow peppers, olives, chopped tomatoes and red onion. Chill well. Season to taste with salt and pepper.

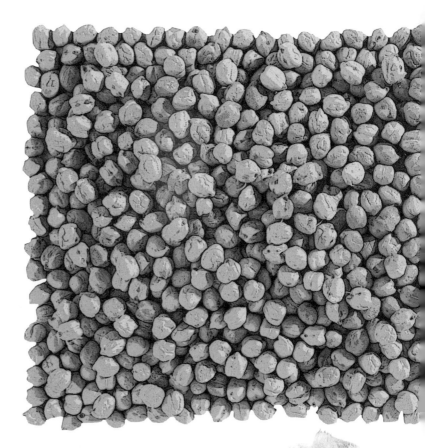

Greek bean and tomato salad

Serves 4 to 6

Vine-ripened tomatoes, arguably the greatest gastronomic pleasure of summer, add the necessary sweetness to this substantial salad. It makes a wonderful lunch or starting course for a dinner, as well as a very useful addition to buffets since it lives nicely for a couple of hours after it's assembled. Feel free to use up to twice as much olive oil as called for in the recipe — that is, if calories aren't a problem — and you'll have a richer taste sensation.

2 cups	cooked white kidney beans or 1 can (19 oz [540 mL]), rinsed and drained	500 mL
2	ripe medium tomatoes, cut into 1/2-inch (1 cm) wedges	2
1/2 cup	thinly sliced red onions	125 mL
4	black olives, pitted and halved	4
	Few sprigs fresh parsley, chopped	
2 tbsp	red wine vinegar	25 mL
2 tbsp	extra virgin olive oil	25 mL
1/2 tsp	salt	2 mL
1/4 tsp	freshly ground black pepper	1 mL
4 oz	feta cheese in big crumbles	125 g
1 tsp	olive oil	5 mL
Half	red bell pepper, cut into thin strips	Half

1. Put beans into a bowl. Add tomatoes, red onions, olives and parsley. Do not toss.

2. In a small bowl, whisk together vinegar, 2 tbsp (25 mL) olive oil, salt and pepper until slightly emulsified. Sprinkle on beans; toss and fold until well mixed, but without mashing beans. Transfer the salad to a serving bowl. Distribute the feta crumbles decoratively on top.

3. In a small frying pan, heat 1 tsp (5 mL) oil over high heat; cook red pepper, turning often, for 3 to 4 minutes or until charred slightly and wilting. Decorate salad with the red peppers. Serve immediately, or cover and keep unrefrigerated for up to 2 hours.

Chili, stews and casseroles

Serves 4

Potato and chickpea stew with spicy sausage

During the long winter months, this is the kind of hearty, legume-based stew with which Southern Europeans bring the sunshine back into their homes. The version we present here is virtually foolproof, requiring just a minimum of attention — and little effort if one uses canned chickpeas (washed with cold running water and strained).

Leftovers are wonderful, since the flavors will intensify upon reheating the next day. It can be enjoyed as a vegetarian main course (just omit the sausages) or you can experiment with substitutes for the sausage; any stewing meat (pork, lamb or chicken) will work well. In all cases, the stew is wonderful if served with a salad and crusty bread.

1/2 cup	red lentils (masoor dal)	125 mL
1 cup	diced peeled potatoes	250 mL
1/2 cup	scraped carrots, cut into 1/4-inch (5 mm) cubes	125 mL
	Boiling water	
1/4 cup	olive oil	50 mL
1 tsp	sweet paprika	5 mL
3/4 tsp	salt	4 mL
1/4 tsp	freshly ground black pepper	1 mL
1/4 tsp	turmeric	1 mL
2 cups	chopped onions	500 mL
1/4 tsp	chili flakes	1 mL
2 tbsp	finely chopped garlic	25 mL
2	medium tomatoes, cut into 1/2-inch (1 cm) wedges	2
2	bay leaves	2
1 tsp	red wine vinegar	5 mL
1/2 tsp	dried oregano	2 mL
1/2 tsp	dried thyme	2 mL
2 cups	cooked chickpeas or 1 can (19 oz [540 mL]) chickpeas, rinsed and drained	500 mL
2	dried figs, cut into 1/4-inch (5 mm) cubes	2
1 lb	spicy sausage (such as merguez, chorizo or spicy Italian)	500 g
2 tbsp	finely minced red onions	25 mL
	Few sprigs fresh parsley, chopped	

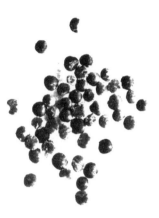

1. Soak lentils in boiling water to cover for 20 minutes; drain. Bring 5 cups (1.25 L) water to a boil; stir in lentils and cook for 5 minutes. Add potatoes and carrots; return to a boil. Reduce heat to medium; cook, stirring very occasionally, for 10 minutes or until the potatoes are tender, but not quite crumbling. Drain, reserving cooking liquid. Set lentils and vegetables aside. Measure out 1 1/2 cups (375 mL) of the cooking liquid and set aside. (If there isn't enough liquid, make up the difference with water.)

2. In a large deep saucepan, heat olive oil over medium-high heat. Add paprika, salt, pepper and turmeric; cook, stirring, for 1 minute, being careful not to let the spices burn. Add onions and chili flakes; cook, stirring, 4 minutes or until the onions are soft and beginning to catch on the bottom of the pan. Add garlic and cook, stirring, for 1 minute. Add tomatoes, bay leaves, vinegar, oregano and thyme; cook, stirring, for 2 to 3 minutes or until tomatoes are starting to break up and a sauce forms.

3. Stir in lentil-vegetable mixture, chickpeas, figs and reserved cooking liquid; bring to a boil. Reduce heat to medium-low and cook for 20 minutes, uncovered, stirring occasionally from the bottom up to avoid scorching. Take off heat, cover and let rest for 10 minutes.

4. While stew rests, grill, broil or fry the sausages. Serve stew garnished with sausages, red onions and parsley.

Cassoulet with pork and zucchini

Serves 6

Baked beans take many forms around the world, and cassoulet is the version favored in the well-fed northern regions of France. There, any number of fatty meats (goose and/or pork fat, for example) are mixed with beans and baked under an equally fatty crust. Here we "Mediterraneanize" the original recipe, using additional vegetables and a lot less fat. Still, this is a hefty and lengthy dish that requires cool weather, a suitable occasion (to justify the effort), and a well-ventilated room.

DEEP BAKING DISH, MEASURING ABOUT
12 BY 16 INCHES (30 BY 40 CM)

1 tbsp	olive oil	15 mL
1/4 tsp	salt	1 mL
1/4 tsp	freshly ground black pepper	1 mL
1 lb	pork tenderloin, cut into 1-inch (2.5 cm) cubes	500 g
1 tbsp	finely chopped garlic	15 mL
1 tbsp	olive oil	15 mL
1/2 tsp	salt	2 mL
1/2 tsp	freshly ground black pepper	2 mL
1 cup	finely diced onions	250 mL
2	medium leeks, trimmed, washed and finely chopped (about 3 cups [750 mL])	2
2	stalks celery with leaves, finely chopped	2
Half	green bell pepper, finely diced	Half
1	large carrot, scraped and finely diced (about 4 oz [125 g])	1
8 oz	mushrooms, trimmed and quartered	250 g
1 lb	tomatoes, peeled and finely chopped (about 2 cups [500 mL]) or canned tomatoes	500 g
1 tbsp	tomato paste, diluted in 1 cup (250 mL) water	15 mL
1 tsp	red wine vinegar	5 mL
1 tsp	dried basil	5 mL
1 tsp	dried oregano	5 mL
2 cups	cooked white kidney beans or 1 can (19 oz [540 mL]), rinsed and drained	500 mL
2 cups	cooked red Romano beans or 1 can (19 oz [540 mL]), rinsed and drained	500 mL
1	medium zucchini, cut into 1/4-inch (5 mm) rounds (about 8 oz [250 g])	1
2 cups	chicken stock	500 mL

Topping

2 cups	breadcrumbs	500 mL
1 tbsp	finely chopped garlic	15 mL
1/2 tsp	ground allspice	2 mL
2	eggs, beaten	2
2 tbsp	olive oil	25 mL
1 cup	dry white vermouth *or* white wine	250 mL
	Few sprigs fresh parsley, chopped	

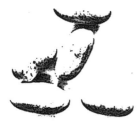

1. In a large nonstick frying pan, heat 1 tbsp (15 mL) olive oil, salt and pepper over high heat for 30 seconds. Add pork and stir-fry for 2 minutes, turning meat often so that all the pieces are thoroughly browned. Add garlic and stir-fry 1 more minute. Transfer contents of the frying pan to a large saucepan.

2. Return the frying pan to high heat. Add 1 tbsp (15 mL) olive oil, salt and pepper; heat for 30 seconds. Add onions, leeks, celery, green pepper, carrot and mushrooms; cook, stirring, for 4 minutes or until the vegetables are softened and a little oily. Transfer vegetables to saucepan with meat.

3. Stir in tomatoes, diluted tomato paste, vinegar, dried basil and oregano. Bring to a boil, cover tightly, reduce heat to medium-low and cook for 25 to 30 minutes or until the meat is cooked through. Remove from heat.

4. Preheat oven to 375° F (190° C). Add white kidney beans, red Romano beans, zucchini and chicken stock to the stew. Gently fold to mix everything thoroughly. Transfer this mixture to baking dish. Spread mixture over bottom of dish, making a layer about 1 1/2 inches (4 cm) deep.

5. Make the topping: In a bowl stir together the breadcrumbs, garlic and allspice until combined. In a small bowl, combine the eggs, olive oil and vermouth. Add this liquid to the breadcrumbs and stir to mix until combined (it'll be wet and lumpy).

6. As evenly as possible, spread this topping over the stew. Bake uncovered for 30 minutes. Remove from oven and press the topping (which will have browned a little) just into the stew, but leaving it still on top. Put back in the oven and bake another 30 minutes or until the topping is nicely crusted and the stew is bubbling underneath.

7. Remove from oven and let rest for 10 minutes. Portion onto plates, keeping breadcrumbs on top; garnish with chopped parsley and serve immediately.

Serves 4 to 6

Beef stew with chorizo and chickpeas

This stew combines French bourguignon technique with the very Spanish flavor of chorizo, whose paprika-garlic essence seems to crop up in just about every kitchen on the Iberian Peninsula.

Strictly speaking, this particular combination is purely an invention of mine; once you've tasted it, however, I'm sure you'll agree it has the savor of a heritage recipe. In any case, this dish certainly has been a big favorite on movie sets I've catered during winter shoots — a tribute, no doubt, to its restorative powers, readying the body for a return to the freezing outdoors for more takes of the beautiful Canadian wilderness.

1/4 cup	olive oil	50 mL
1/4 tsp	freshly ground black pepper	1 mL
1 1/2 lbs	lean stewing beef, cut into 3/4-inch (2 cm) cubes	750 g
8 oz	chorizo sausage, cut into 1/2-inch (1 cm) pieces	250 g
2 tbsp	finely chopped garlic	25 mL
1 tsp	sweet paprika	5 mL
1 cup	red wine	250 mL
1 cup	chicken stock	250 mL
2 tbsp	tomato paste, diluted in 1/2 cup (125 mL) water	25 mL
1 tsp	dried oregano	5 mL
2	bay leaves	2
1	potato, peeled and cut into 1/2-inch (1 cm) cubes (about 1 cup [250 mL])	1
2 cups	cooked chickpeas or 1 can (19 oz [540 mL]), rinsed and drained	500 mL
1/2 cup	finely diced red onions	125 mL
	Steamed rice as an accompaniment	
	Few sprigs fresh coriander or parsley, chopped	

1. In a large nonstick frying pan, heat olive oil and pepper over high heat for 1 minute. Add the beef and the chorizo (in batches if necessary) and fry, turning often, for 2 to 3 minutes or until the beef is thoroughly seared and the chorizo is sizzling. Transfer the meat to a saucepan, leaving as much of the oil as possible in the frying pan.

2. Return frying pan to high heat. Add garlic and paprika; stir-fry for 1 minute or until starting to brown. Add wine; bring to a boil, stirring. Add chicken stock and diluted tomato paste; keep stirring and bring to a boil. Pour this sauce and all its bits over the meat.

3. Stir in oregano, bay leaves and potato. Bring stew to a boil; reduce heat to medium-low, cover tightly and cook, stirring once every 15 minutes to avoid scorching, for 1 hour (mild bubbles throughout) or until the meat and potatoes are tender.

4. Stir in chickpeas; cook uncovered for 5 to 7 minutes. Stir, cover and remove from heat. Let rest for 10 minutes, then portion it alongside rice and garnish with red onions and fresh coriander. Serve immediately.

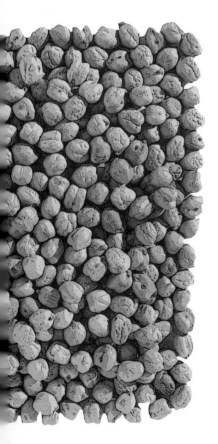

Make-ahead southwestern pork stew

Serves 6

Here's a soothing dish to serve for casual get-togethers. This stew requires no more preparation time than a stir-fry or one-pot dish. Cutting the meat into smaller pieces also shortens the cooking time.

Tip

Lean stewing beef can be substituted for the pork. For a vegetarian dish, replace meat with cubes of firm tofu. Add along with kidney beans.

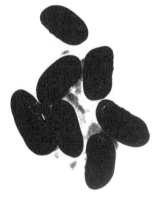

4 tsp	olive oil	20 mL
1 lb	lean stewing pork, cut into 3/4-inch (2 cm) cubes	500 g
2	medium onions, chopped	2
3	cloves garlic, finely chopped	3
4 tsp	chili powder	20 mL
1 1/2 tsp	dried oregano	7 mL
1 tsp	ground cumin	5 mL
3/4 tsp	salt	4 mL
1/2 tsp	red pepper flakes	2 mL
3 tbsp	all-purpose flour	45 mL
2 cups	beef stock *or* chicken stock	500 mL
1	can (28 oz [796 mL]) tomatoes, chopped	1
2	bell peppers (assorted colors), cubed	2
2 cups	frozen corn kernels	500 mL
1	can (19 oz [540 mL]) kidney beans or black beans, rinsed and drained	1
	Chopped coriander (optional)	

1. In a large Dutch oven, heat half the oil over high heat; brown pork in batches. Transfer to a plate. Add remaining oil to pan; reduce heat to medium. Add onions, garlic, chili powder, oregano, cumin, salt and red pepper flakes; cook, stirring, for 2 minutes or until softened.

2. Sprinkle with flour; stir in stock and tomatoes. Bring to a boil, stirring until thickened. Return pork and accumulated juices to pan; reduce heat, cover and simmer for 1 hour or until meat is tender.

3. Add bell peppers, corn and kidney beans; simmer, covered, for 15 minutes or until vegetables are tender. Garnish with chopped coriander, if desired.

Pork and black bean stew with sweet potatoes

This is a gorgeous stew — tender pieces of boneless pork, highlighted by shiny black beans and cubes of deep orange sweet potatoes. A sprinkling of chopped cilantro just before serving adds real Western flavor and even more bright color to the mix. I like this healthy combination served with a mound of creamy mashed potatoes or cornbread.

To save time, use canned black beans, rinsed and drained.

PREHEAT OVEN TO 350° F (180° C)
12-CUP (3 L) CASSEROLE DISH WITH LID

2 tbsp	olive oil	25 mL
4 lbs	boneless pork shoulder, cut into 1-inch (2.5 cm) cubes	2 kg
2 tbsp	all-purpose flour	25 mL
2	sweet potatoes (about 1 lb [500 g]), peeled and cubed	2
1 1/2 cups	chicken stock	375 mL
1 1/2 cups	chopped onions	375 mL
1 cup	dry white wine	250 mL
1/2 cup	chopped fresh parsley	125 mL
1/4 cup	red wine vinegar	50 mL
6	cloves garlic, minced	6
1 tbsp	ground cumin	15 mL
2 cups	cooked black beans	500 mL
1 tsp	ground cumin	5 mL
1/2 tsp	freshly ground black pepper	2 mL
1/2 cup	chopped cilantro	125 mL

1. In a large frying pan, heat oil over medium-high heat. In batches, cook pork, turning occasionally, for 5 minutes or until browned. Transfer pork to casserole dish as it is browned.

2. Sprinkle flour over the pork and toss. Add the sweet potatoes, chicken stock, onions, wine, parsley, vinegar, half of the garlic and 1 tbsp (15 mL) cumin; mix well. Cover and bake for 1 hour.

3. Stir in beans, 1 tsp (5 mL) cumin, pepper and remaining garlic. Bake, uncovered, for 15 minutes or until slightly thickened. Just before serving, stir in the cilantro.

Prairie fire beans

Serves 10

Dried beans keep indefinitely and, when eaten with rice or other grains, are a complete protein — high in fiber and complex carbohydrates, as well as low in fat.

In Texas and Mexico, red beans or mottled pinto beans are most common and are the basis for most chili dishes. Further north, the Great Northern bean is grown. This large white bean is the North American version of the Haricot bean or Italian Cannellini bean. Navy or pea beans are smaller white beans, used for pots of molasses-spiked baked beans or in soups. Heirloom beans like Tongues of Fire, Anasazi, flageolots and Rattlesnakes have taken on a new cachet as today's western cooks search for healthier ways to cut down on fat and protein in their traditionally meat-based diets.

2 lbs	dried pinto beans (about 5 cups [1.25 L]), soaked overnight in water to cover	1 kg
1	large ham hock or ham bone	1
1	small whole onion, peeled	1
Pinch	salt	Pinch
2 tbsp	butter	25 mL
1 lb	sharp Cheddar cheese, shredded	500 g
1 tsp	Prairie Fire hot sauce or other hot sauce	5 mL
1 cup	finely chopped onions	250 mL
2	cloves garlic, minced	2
	Additional hot sauce to taste	
	Salt and pepper to taste	

1. In a large saucepan, combine drained beans, ham hock, whole onion and a pinch of salt. Add cold water to cover beans by 2 inches (5 cm). Bring to a boil, reduce heat to low and simmer, covered, for 1 hour or until beans are tender.

2. Discard ham hock and onion. Drain beans; return to saucepan. Stir in butter, cheese, hot sauce, onions and garlic. Cook, covered, over low heat for 20 minutes or until cheese melts and everything is tender.

3. Season to taste with additional hot sauce, salt and pepper.

Greek chili with black olives and feta cheese

Serves 4

Tip
Leave the skin on zucchini and eggplant for extra fiber.

Other canned beans can be used, such as chickpeas, navy white beans or black beans.

Another cheese can replace feta, such as goat, Cheddar or mozzarella.

Make Ahead
Prepare up to a day ahead and gently reheat, adding more stock if too thick.

Great as leftovers.

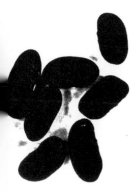

1 tsp	vegetable oil	5 mL
2 tsp	minced garlic	10 mL
1 cup	chopped onions	250 mL
1 cup	chopped zucchini	250 mL
1 cup	sliced mushrooms	250 mL
1 cup	chopped green bell peppers	250 mL
1 1/2 cups	chopped eggplant	375 mL
8 oz	lean ground beef or lamb	250 g
1	can (19 oz [540 mL]) tomatoes, puréed	1
1 1/2 cups	beef or chicken stock	375 mL
1 cup	canned red kidney beans, drained	250 mL
1 cup	canned white kidney beans, drained	250 mL
1/3 cup	sliced black olives	75 mL
1 tbsp	chili powder	15 mL
1 1/2 tsp	dried basil	7 mL
1 1/2 tsp	dried oregano	7 mL
2 oz	feta cheese, crumbled	50 g

1. In a large nonstick saucepan sprayed with vegetable spray, heat oil over medium heat. Add garlic, onions, zucchini, mushrooms, green peppers and eggplant; cook for 8 minutes or until softened. Add beef and cook, stirring to break up, for 2 minutes or until no longer pink. Drain any excess fat.
2. Mash 1/2 cup (125 mL) of the red kidney beans and 1/2 cup (125 mL) of the white kidney beans. Add tomatoes, stock, mashed and whole beans, olives, chili powder, basil and oregano to saucepan; bring to a boil. Reduce heat to low and simmer, covered, for 30 minutes. Sprinkle with cheese before serving.

Serves 10 to 12

Northern bounty baked beans

Baked beans — real baked beans — make one of the best partners with grilled fare. The finest ever were served up at the first Northern Bounty, a now bi-annual food conference organized by Cuisine Canada, the national organi-zation that keeps the Canadian culinary scene in sharp focus. These are Calgary cowboy-style baked beans, slow-cooked with salt pork, molasses and pure maple syrup. These are sim-ply the best — there's noth-ing better with ribs, creamy coleslaw and corn.

BEAN POT OR HEAVY CASSEROLE WITH LID

4 cups	dried white navy beans	1 L
10 cups	cold water	2.5 L
1 lb	salt pork, sliced	500 g
2	onions, minced	2
1/2 cup	tomato paste	125 mL
1/2 cup	brown sugar	125 mL
1/2 cup	pure maple syrup	125 mL
1 tbsp	dry mustard	15 mL
1/3 cup	fancy molasses	75 mL

1. Place beans in a colander; wash thoroughly and remove any stones. Place in a large pot with cold water. Soak overnight.

2. Preheat oven to 325° F (160° C). Place beans over high heat; bring to a boil. Reduce heat; simmer gently, cov-ered, for 30 minutes or until tender.

3. Line the inside of bean pot or casserole with salt pork. Set aside.

4. Add onions, tomato paste, brown sugar, maple syrup, mustard and molasses to beans. Stir to blend well. Pour carefully into pork-lined bean pot. Cover; bake, stirring occasionally, in preheated oven for 4 to 4 1/2 hours or until beans are tender and sauce has thick-ened. Add water if necessary. Remove from heat; dis-card pork slices before serving.

Amazing chili

Serves 6 to 8

Every cook has a special version of chili. Here's mine — it's meaty and nicely spiced with just the right amount of beans. Not everyone agrees that beans belong in a chili — witness the Texas version dubbed "bowl of red" — but I love the way the beans absorb the spices and rich tomato flavor.

Tip

The flavor of the chili hinges on the quality of chili powder used. Most powders are a blend of dried, ground mild chilies, as well as cumin, oregano, garlic and salt.

Read the list of ingredients to be sure you're not buying one with starch and sugar fillers. Chili powder should not be confused with powdered or ground chilies of the cayenne pepper variety.

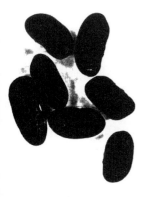

1 1/2 lbs	lean ground beef	750 g
2	medium onions, chopped	2
3	cloves garlic, finely chopped	3
2	stalks celery, chopped	2
1	large green bell pepper, chopped	1
2 tbsp	chili powder	25 mL
1 1/2 tsp	dried oregano	7 mL
1 1/2 tsp	ground cumin	7 mL
1 tsp	salt	5 mL
1/2 tsp	red pepper flakes, or to taste	2 mL
1	can (28 oz [796 mL]) tomatoes, chopped, juice reserved	1
1 cup	beef stock	250 mL
1	can (19 oz [540 mL]) pinto or red kidney beans, drained and rinsed	1
1/4 cup	chopped fresh parsley or coriander	50 mL

1. In a Dutch oven, brown beef over medium-high heat, breaking up with back of a spoon, for about 7 minutes or until no longer pink.
2. Reduce heat to medium. Add onions, garlic, celery, green pepper, chili powder, oregano, cumin, salt and red pepper flakes; cook, stirring often, for 5 minutes or until vegetables are softened.
3. Stir in the tomatoes with juice and the stock. Bring to a boil; reduce heat, cover and simmer, stirring occasionally, for 1 hour.
4. Add beans and parsley; cover and simmer for 10 minutes more.

Molasses baked beans

Serves 8

Here's an old-time favorite that stirs memories of the pioneer spirit. This rustic dish is a winter standby and wonderful when served with home-baked bread.

Tip

For a vegetarian version, omit bacon and cook onions and garlic in 2 tbsp (25 mL) vegetable oil.

PREHEAT OVEN TO 300° F (150° C)
12-CUP (3 L) CASSEROLE DISH OR BEAN POT

1 lb	dried Great Northern or white pea beans (about 2 1/4 cups [550 mL]), rinsed and picked over	500 g
6	slices lean smoky bacon, chopped	6
1	large onion, chopped	1
3	cloves garlic, finely chopped	3
1	can (7 1/2 oz [213 mL]) tomato sauce	1
1/3 cup	molasses	75 mL
1/4 cup	packed brown sugar	50 mL
2 tbsp	balsamic vinegar	25 mL
2 tsp	dry mustard	10 mL
1 tsp	salt	5 mL
1/4 tsp	pepper	1 mL

1. In a Dutch oven, combine beans with 6 cups (1.5 L) cold water. Bring to a boil over high heat; boil for 2 minutes. Remove from heat, cover and let stand for 1 hour.

2. Drain beans and cover with 8 cups (2 L) cold water; bring to a boil. Reduce heat and simmer, covered, for 30 to 40 minutes or until beans are just tender but still hold their shape. Drain, reserving 2 cups (500 mL) cooking liquid. Place beans in casserole dish or bean pot.

3. Meanwhile, in a saucepan, cook bacon over medium heat, stirring often, for 5 minutes or until crisp. Drain all but 2 tbsp (25 mL) fat in pan. Add onion and garlic; cook, stirring, for 3 minutes or until softened.

4. Add 2 cups (500 mL) reserved bean-cooking liquid, tomato sauce, molasses, brown sugar, balsamic vinegar, mustard, salt and pepper. Stir into beans.

5. Cover and bake in preheated oven for 2 1/2 to 3 hours or until most of liquid has been absorbed.

Serves 4 to 6

20-minute chili

Here's a streamlined version of chili that's a snap. Make a double batch and have containers stashed away in the freezer for quick microwave meals. Just ladle into bowls and, if desired, top with shredded Monterey Jack cheese. Set out a basket of crusty bread — supper is that easy.

Tip
Add just a pinch of red pepper flakes for a mild chili; but if you want to turn up the heat, use amount specified in the recipe.

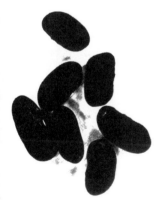

1 lb	lean ground beef or turkey	500 g
1	large onion, chopped	1
2	large cloves garlic, finely chopped	2
1	large green bell pepper, chopped	1
4 tsp	chili powder	20 mL
1 tbsp	all-purpose flour	15 mL
1 tsp	dried basil	5 mL
1 tsp	dried oregano	5 mL
1/4 to 1/2 tsp	red pepper flakes	1 to 2 mL
2 cups	tomato pasta sauce	500 mL
1 1/3 cups	beef stock	325 mL
1	can (19 oz [540 mL]) kidney beans or pinto beans, rinsed and drained	1
	Salt and pepper	

1. In a Dutch oven or large saucepan over medium-high heat, cook beef, breaking up with a wooden spoon, for 5 minutes or until no longer pink.
2. Reduce heat to medium. Add onion, garlic, green pepper, chili powder, flour, basil, oregano and red pepper flakes; cook, stirring, for 4 minutes or until vegetables are softened. Stir in tomato sauce and stock. Bring to a boil; cook, stirring, until thickened. Add beans; season with salt and pepper to taste. Reduce heat and simmer, covered, for 10 minutes.

Wagon boss chili

Serves 6

This chili is served at an Alberta guest ranch, where you can recall the days of the big cattle drives, complete with thousands of head of cattle and mounted cowboys, led by the wagon boss.

When cowboy cooks first put meat and peppers together, the seeds of modern-day chili were sown and the West became the official domain of chili, hot sauces, searing salsas and chiliheads.

Substitute Romano beans or red kidney beans if you can't find pinto beans.

2 tbsp	canola oil	25 mL
2 lbs	lean round steak, cut into 1/2-inch (1 cm) cubes	1 kg
3	cloves garlic, minced	3
2 cups	chopped onions	500 mL
2 cups	beef broth	500 mL
2 cups	canned tomatoes with juices, chopped	500 mL
2 tbsp	chili powder	25 mL
1 tsp	dried oregano	5 mL
1 tsp	ground cumin	5 mL
1/2 tsp	cayenne pepper	2 mL
1/2 tsp	salt	2 mL
1/4 tsp	freshly ground black pepper	1 mL
1	can (19 oz [540 mL]) pinto beans, rinsed and drained	1
3 tbsp	cornmeal	45 mL

1. In a Dutch oven, heat oil over medium-high heat. In several batches, cook beef, turning occasionally, for 5 minutes or until well-browned. Return all beef to saucepan, along with garlic and onions; cook for 5 minutes or until onions are tender.

2. Stir in 1 cup (250 mL) water, beef broth, tomatoes, chili powder, oregano, cumin, cayenne pepper, salt and pepper. Bring to a boil, reduce heat to low and simmer, covered, for 2 hours or until meat is very tender.

3. Stir in beans and cornmeal; simmer for another 20 minutes or until mixture is heated through and thickened.

Serves 8

Dutch ovens are cast iron pots that can be suspended above the fire or set right down into the fire on their stubby legs and surrounded by coals. More coals are piled on the lids and the ovens left to "bake" their contents, whether they be biscuits, roasts or loaves of bread.

Cooking over a campfire in a Dutch oven is not easy. Many cowboy cooks report campfire cooking disasters, from charred biscuit and scorched stews to petrified eggs, coming from these big cast iron pots. The best advice, says one cook, is to use good hardwood to build your fire. Oak, hickory, maple or mesquite will all provide good heat-holding coals for hours of cooking while soft woods like cedar, aspen or poplar make for poor, inconsistent heat and bitter smoke.

Pork and beef chili with ancho sauce

2	dried ancho chilies	2
1/4 cup	olive oil	50 mL
1 lb	pork shoulder stew meat, cut into 1/2-inch (1 cm) cubes	500 g
1 lb	beef chuck steak, cut into 1/4- to 1/2-inch (5 mm to 1 cm) cubes	500 g
1	large onion, chopped	1
5	cloves garlic, minced	5
4 oz	spicy Italian sausage, casings removed	125 g
1 tbsp	ground cumin	15 mL
1 tbsp	crushed hot chilies	15 mL
2	cans (each 19 oz [540 mL]) tomatoes, chopped	2
1/4 cup	rye whisky	50 mL
1 tbsp	dried oregano	15 mL
1 1/2 cups	cooked black beans	375 mL
1/4 cup	tomato paste	50 mL
	Salt and pepper to taste	

1. Soak ancho chilies in hot water 20 minutes or until softened; drain. Chop, discarding stems and seeds; set aside.

2. In a large Dutch oven, heat oil over medium-high heat. In several batches, cook diced pork and beef, turning often, for 4 minutes or until well-browned. With a slotted spoon, transfer to a bowl leaving behind as much oil as possible; set aside. Reduce heat to medium-low. Add onion, garlic and sausage; cook, stirring to break up meat, for 4 minutes or until onion is softened and meat is no longer pink. Stir in ancho chilies, cumin and crushed chilies; cook for 5 minutes or until onion is tender.

3. Stir in browned pork and beef, tomatoes, whisky and oregano. Bring to a boil. Reduce heat to low and simmer, covered, for 1 1/2 hours.

4. Stir in beans and tomato paste. Simmer 15 minutes longer to heat through. Season to taste with salt and pepper.

Prairie bean cassoulet

Serves 8

Beans from Taber, Alberta, combined with lamb and old-fashioned Ukrainian or Italian sausage are featured in this simplified prairie version of a traditional French dish. Enjoy it after a day of skiing, served with lots of mashed potatoes.

After Step 2, layer the beans, meat mixture and sausage in a slow cooker, adding liquid as necessary. Cook on low heat for 12 hours. Turn cassoulet into casserole dish and proceed with Step 4.

14-CUP (3.5 L) BEAN POT, CASSEROLE DISH OR ROASTING PAN

1 lb	dried navy beans (about 2 1/4 cups [550 mL]), rinsed	500 g
8 oz	bacon (preferably double-smoked), chopped	250 g
1 tsp	coarse salt	5 mL
1 tsp	chopped fresh thyme	5 mL
1 tsp	chopped fresh rosemary	5 mL
1 tsp	freshly ground black pepper	5 mL
2	cloves garlic, minced	2
2 tbsp	canola oil	25 mL
1 1/2 lbs	lamb or pork shoulder, cut into 1-inch (2.5 cm) cubes	750 g
1 cup	chopped onions	250 mL
1	ripe tomato, chopped	1
2 tbsp	tomato paste	25 mL
1/2 tsp	ground cloves	2 mL
1 lb	kielbasa *or* Italian sausage	500 g

Topping

1 cup	dry bread crumbs	250 mL
1/4 cup	melted butter	50 mL
2 tbsp	chopped fresh parsley	25 mL
1/2 tsp	freshly ground black pepper	2 mL
2	cloves garlic, minced	2

(Recipe continues...)

AMAZING CHILI (PAGE 91) ➤

OVERLEAF: MAPLE BAKED PORK AND BEANS WITH CARAMELIZED APPLES (PAGE 98)

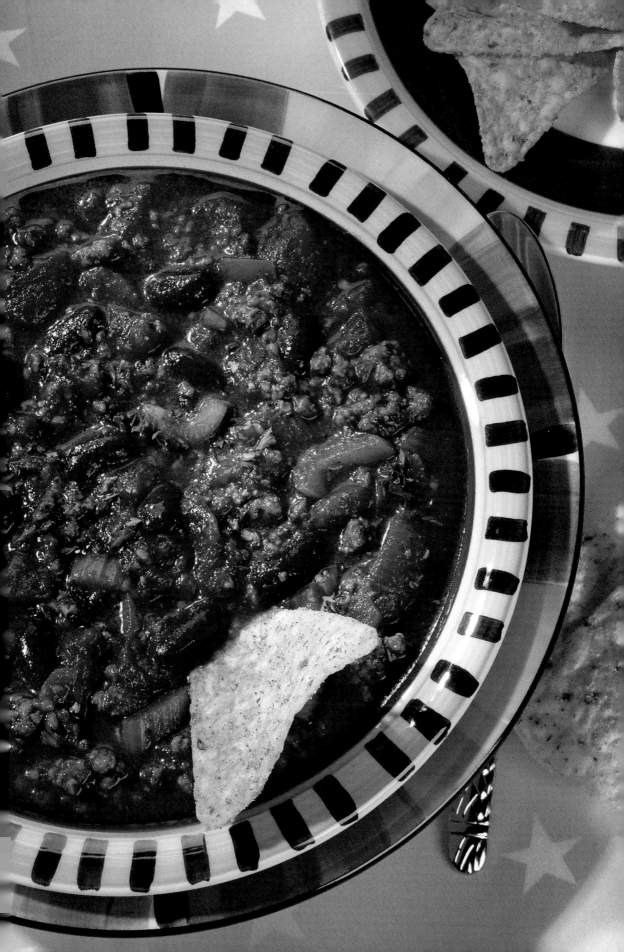

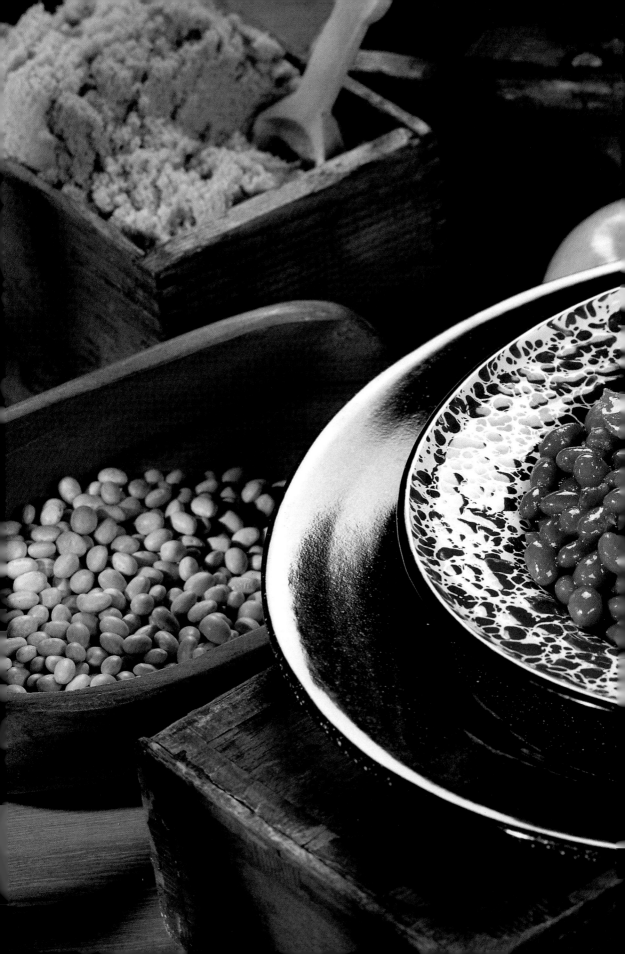

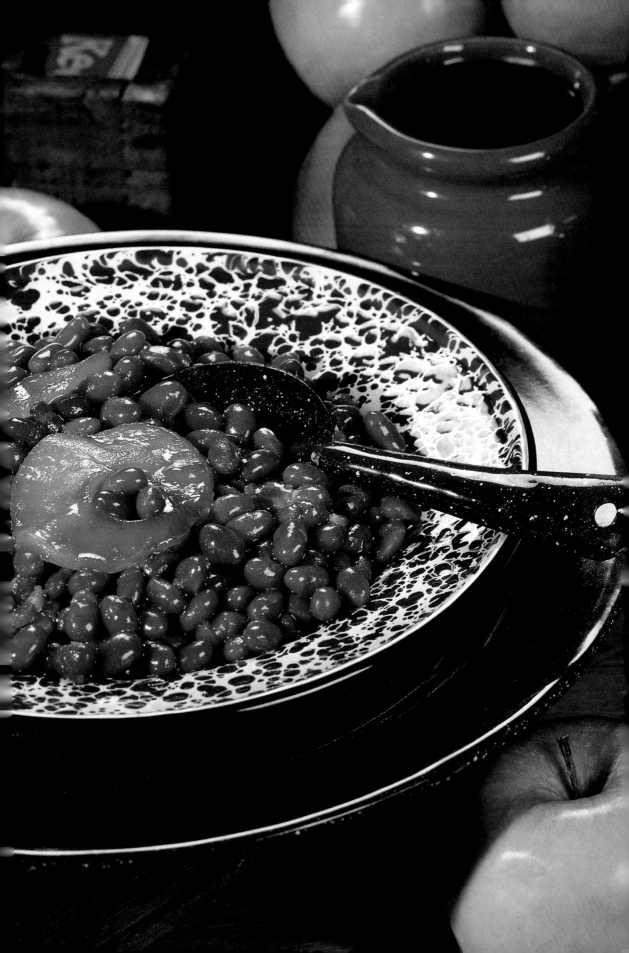

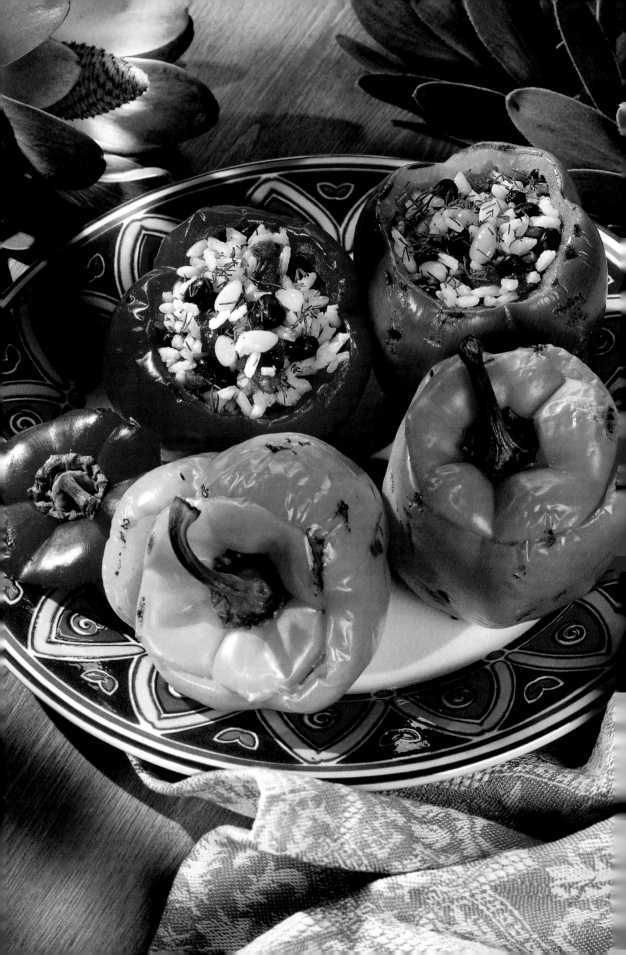

1. In a large saucepan, combine beans and 3 cups (750 mL) water; bring to a boil. Remove from heat; let stand, covered, for 40 minutes. Drain. Put half of the bacon in the bottom of the saucepan; top with drained beans. Add salt and 4 cups (1 L) of water. Bring to a boil, reduce heat to low and simmer, covered, for 1 1/2 hours or until tender. Drain beans, reserving cooking liquid. Set beans and bean cooking liquid aside.

2. Meanwhile, mix the thyme, rosemary, pepper and garlic; rub over the cubed lamb or pork. In a large frying pan, heat oil over medium-high heat; in batches, cook meat, turning occasionally, for 5 minutes or until well browned. With a slotted spoon, transfer meat to a bowl, leaving behind as much oil as possible. Cook remaining bacon and onions for 4 minutes or until onions are translucent. Stir in browned meat, tomato, tomato paste and cloves; set aside.

3. In a nonstick frying pan sprayed with vegetable spray, cook Italian sausage, if using, over medium-high heat, turning occasionally, for 5 minutes or until browned. Cut kielbasa or browned Italian sausage into chunks; set aside.

4. Preheat oven to 300° F (150° C). In roasting pan, layer one-third of the beans, one-third of the meat mixture and one-third of the sausage; repeat layers twice. Add just enough of the bean cooking liquid to come to the top layer of beans, adding extra water if necessary. Bake, covered, for 2 hours or until meat is tender. Remove from oven. Increase oven heat to 350° F (180° C).

5. In a bowl stir together bread crumbs, butter, parsley, pepper and garlic. Sprinkle over cassoulet. Bake, uncovered, for 20 minutes or until topping is golden brown.

≺ RICE AND BLACK BEAN STUFFED PEPPERS (PAGE 130)

Maple baked pork and beans with caramelized apples

Serves 8

This recipe makes a delicious old-fashioned bean dish, good alongside your barbecue beef on a bun — or even with pancakes — for a Stampede breakfast. It's a variation of a recipe Calgarian Rick Gauthier entered in a bean contest and for which he won second place.

12-CUP (3 L) BEAN POT OR CASSEROLE DISH

2 cups	dried navy beans, rinsed	500 mL
1 tbsp	molasses	15 mL
8 oz	back bacon, preferably double-smoked	250 g
4	Granny Smith apples	4
1	large onion, chopped	1
1/2 cup	maple syrup	125 mL
1 tbsp	dry mustard	15 mL
1 tsp	coarse salt	5 mL
1/4 cup	butter	50 mL
1/4 cup	packed brown sugar	50 mL
1/2 cup	rum	125 mL

1. In a saucepan combine beans, molasses and 8 cups (2 L) water; bring to a boil. Remove from heat; let stand, covered, for 1 hour. Uncover. Bring to a boil, reduce heat to low and simmer, covered, for 45 minutes to 1 hour or until beans are starting to get tender. Drain.

2. Preheat oven to 325° F (160° C). Chop bacon into thin slivers. Peel and chop 2 of the apples. In a bean pot, combine drained beans, bacon, chopped apples, onion, maple syrup, mustard and salt. Cover and bake for 3 hours. Stir; if beans seem dry, add a little hot water. Cover and bake 1 to 2 hours longer.

3. Meanwhile, core remaining apples and slice into 1/2-inch (1 cm) rings. In a frying pan, melt butter over medium heat. Stir in brown sugar; cook for 2 minutes, stirring occasionally. Add apple rings, stirring to coat with sugar. Add half of the rum; increase heat to medium-high and cook, turning rings occasionally, for 8 minutes or until the liquid evaporates and apples are tender. Set aside.

4. Remove cover from bean pot and arrange caramelized apple slices on top of the beans. Bake, uncovered, for 30 minutes. Just before serving, pour the remaining rum slowly over the beans.

Black bean chili

Serves 4 to 6

Tip

Serve this robust chili over baked sweet or regular potatoes for a main dish or with whole grain nachos for an appetizer or party dish.

Because many of the water-soluble nutrients are in the canned liquid, try to use both the beans and the liquid from the tin. When cooking fresh beans, however, do not use cooking liquid.

Variations

Substitute: 2 cups (500 mL) any cooked beans.

2 tbsp	olive oil	25 mL
1 cup	chopped onions	250 mL
3	cloves garlic, minced	3
1 1/2 cups	chopped red bell peppers	375 mL
2	whole chilies, crushed	2
2 tsp	ground cumin	10 mL
1	can (28 oz [796 mL]) tomatoes with juice	1
1	can (19 oz [540 mL]) black beans, with liquid	1
1	can (19 oz [540 mL]) chickpeas, with liquid	1
2 tbsp	dried thyme leaves	25 mL
1 tbsp	dried savory leaves	15 mL
2 tbsp	fresh chopped parsley	25 mL

1. In a large skillet, heat oil over medium heat. Add onions, garlic, peppers and chilies; cook for 5 minutes or until soft.
2. Stir in cumin, tomatoes, black beans, chickpeas, thyme and savory. Bring to a boil; simmer for 5 minutes. Stir in parsley and serve.

Chickpea tofu stew

Serves 4

A filling and flavorful winter dish, this stew is bolstered with the addition of the super-nutritious tofu. It is imperative to use firm tofu (often called "pressed tofu"), since the soft variety will disintegrate. For chickpeas, you can either cook your own, or use the canned variety.

Excellent served with a salad, steamed rice and a yogurt-based sauce.

For a spicier flavor, substitute cayenne pepper for the chili powder.

PREHEAT OVEN TO 375° F (190° C)
6-CUP (1.5 L) CASSEROLE DISH

1 lb	ripe tomatoes (about 4)	500 g
3 tbsp	olive oil	45 mL
1/2 tsp	salt	2 mL
1/2 tsp	paprika	2 mL
1/2 tsp	whole cumin seeds	2 mL
1/2 tsp	chili powder	2 mL
2 1/2 cups	thinly sliced onions	625 mL
Half	green bell pepper, thinly sliced	Half
4	cloves garlic, thinly sliced	4
2	bay leaves	2
1 cup	hot water	250 mL
2 tsp	lime juice	10 mL
2 cups	cooked chickpeas	500 mL
8 oz	firm tofu, cut into 1/2-inch (1 cm) cubes	250 g
1 tsp	olive oil (optional)	5 mL
1/4 cup	finely diced red onions	50 mL
	Few sprigs fresh coriander, chopped	

1. Blanch tomatoes in boiling water for 30 seconds. Over a bowl, peel, core and deseed them. Chop tomatoes into chunks and set aside. Strain any accumulated tomato juices from bowl; add the juices to the tomatoes.

2. In a large frying pan, heat olive oil over high heat for 30 seconds. Add salt, paprika, cumin seeds and chili powder in quick succession. Stir-fry for 30 seconds. Add onions and stir-fry for 1 minute. Add green pepper and stir-fry for 2 to 3 minutes or until soft. Add garlic and stir-fry for 1 minute. Add the tomato flesh and juices. Cook, stirring, for 3 minutes, breaking up the tomato somewhat. Add the bay leaves, hot water and lime juice. Cook, stirring often, for 5 minutes.

3. Transfer sauce to casserole dish. Fold the chickpeas into the sauce. Distribute the tofu cubes evenly over the surface, and gently press them down into the sauce.

4. Bake the stew, uncovered, for 25 to 30 minutes, until bubbling and bright. Drizzle with olive oil (if using) and garnish with red onions and coriander.

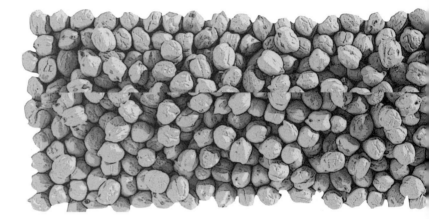

Romano bean stew

Serves 4 to 6

Lovers of hot food will enjoy this combination of spicy sauce, sweetly plump romano beans and fried almonds. It is best served with other spicy dishes, but it works wonderfully to perk up simple meals of rice and plain vegetables. For romano beans you can either cook your own, or use canned. A 19-ounce (540 mL) can of romano beans, rinsed and drained, will yield exactly 2 cups (500 mL), which you'll need for this recipe.

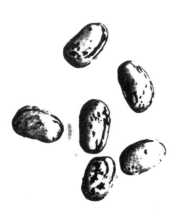

2	medium tomatoes	2
1/4 cup	olive oil	50 mL
1/2 tsp	salt	2 mL
1 tsp	whole cumin seeds	5 mL
2	onions, sliced	2
1	fresh jalapeño pepper, diced (with or without seeds, depending on desired hotness)	1
1/2 cup	water	125 mL
1 tbsp	raisins	15 mL
2 cups	cooked romano beans	500 mL
1 tbsp	olive oil	15 mL
1/2 cup	slivered almonds	125 mL

1. Blanch tomatoes in boiling water for 30 seconds. Over a bowl, peel, core and deseed them. Chop tomatoes into chunks and set aside. Strain any accumulated tomato juices from bowl; add the juices to the tomatoes.

2. In a deep frying pan, heat olive oil over high heat for 1 minute. Add salt and cumin seeds and stir-fry for 1 minute. Add onions and stir-fry for 2 minutes or until softened. Add jalapeño pepper (and seeds, if desired). Stir-fry for 1 to 2 minutes or until ingredients are well coated and starting to char.

3. Add reserved tomato and juices. Stir-fry for 2 to 3 minutes until tomatoes are breaking up. Add water and let it come back to a boil. Stir in raisins, then fold in beans. Reduce heat to medium-low and simmer for 5 minutes, stirring occasionally to prevent scorching. Transfer to a serving bowl.

4. In a frying pan, heat oil over high heat for 30 seconds. Add slivered almonds and fry for 1 to 2 minutes, stirring and turning constantly until browned. Take off heat and immediately transfer to a cool dish. Scatter the almonds on top of the beans. This dish will be at its best if allowed to rest for 1 or 2 hours, then served at room temperature.

Serves 6

Bean and sweet potato chili on garlic polenta

Tip
Use any cooked beans that you have on hand.

Try fresh fennel instead of leeks.

Polenta is delicious, nutritious and takes minutes to make.

A great source of fiber.

Make Ahead
Prepare chili up to 2 days in advance. Cook polenta just before serving.

Chili

2 tsp	vegetable oil	10 mL
1 1/2 tsp	minced garlic	7 mL
1 1/2 cups	chopped leeks	375 mL
1 cup	chopped red bell peppers	250 mL
1	can (19 oz [540 mL]) tomatoes, puréed	1
1 1/2 cups	canned red kidney beans, rinsed and drained	375 mL
1 1/4 cups	chopped peeled sweet potatoes	300 mL
1 tbsp	fennel seeds	15 mL
2 tsp	chili powder	10 mL
1 tsp	dried basil	5 mL

Polenta

3 1/4 cups	vegetable stock	800 mL
1 cup	cornmeal	250 mL
1 tsp	minced garlic	5 mL

1. In a large nonstick saucepan, heat oil over medium-high heat. Add garlic, leeks and red peppers; cook 4 minutes or until softened. Stir in tomatoes, beans, sweet potatoes, fennel seeds, chili powder and basil; bring to a boil. Reduce heat to medium-low and cook, covered, for 20 to 25 minutes or until sweet potatoes are tender.

2. Meanwhile, in a deep saucepan, bring vegetable stock to a boil. Reduce heat to low and gradually whisk in cornmeal and garlic. Cook 5 minutes, stirring frequently.

3. Pour polenta into a serving dish. Spoon chili over top. Serve immediately.

Vegetarian chili

Serves 6 to 8

This recipe comes from a café in Calgary called The Breadline. It's easy to make and chock full of healthy vegetables. Although you probably won't find many vegetarian cowboys, this is a very tasty chili, very low in fat, and excellent as a meatless dinner or side dish.

1/3 cup	olive oil	75 mL
1 lb	zucchini, cut into 1/2-inch (1 cm) dice	500 g
1 lb	onions, cut into 1/2-inch (1 cm) dice	500 g
4	cloves garlic, minced	4
1	large red bell pepper, chopped	1
2	cans (each 28 oz [796 mL]) tomatoes, crushed	2
1 1/2 lbs	cubed ripe tomatoes (about 4 cups [1 L] chopped)	750 g
4 tsp	chili powder	20 mL
1 tbsp	ground cumin	15 mL
1 tbsp	dried basil	15 mL
1 tbsp	dried oregano	15 mL
1 1/2 tsp	freshly ground pepper	7 mL
1 tsp	salt	5 mL
1 tsp	fennel seed	5 mL
2 tbsp	chopped fresh parsley	25 mL
1	can (19 oz [540 mL]) red kidney beans, rinsed and drained	1
1	can (14 oz [398 mL]) chickpeas, rinsed and drained	1
1 tbsp	chopped fresh dill	15 mL
1 tbsp	lemon juice	15 mL
3/4 tsp	granulated sugar	4 mL

1. In a large saucepan, heat olive oil over medium-high heat. Add zucchini, onions, garlic and pepper; cook, stirring often, for 8 minutes or until starting to soften. Stir in canned and fresh tomatoes, chili powder, cumin, basil, oregano, pepper, salt, fennel seed and parsley; bring to a boil. Reduce heat to medium and simmer, uncovered and stirring often, for 30 minutes.

2. Stir in kidney beans, chickpeas, dill, lemon juice and sugar; cook for 15 minutes.

Meat, poultry and fish

Braised stuffed bean curd

Serves 4 to 5

Bean curd (dofu in Chinese or tofu in Japanese) is a cooked, solid form of soybean milk that has been used in Chinese cookery for at least 2,000 years and has spread throughout East and Southeast Asia. It is bland by nature and therefore acts as a good background for tasty sauces. Although it is very important as a protein source for vegetarians — in North America it is almost synonymous with vegetarian food — Asians often cook bean curd with meat or fish. It helps a small amount of meat go a long way.

In this Chinese dish, the bean curd is stuffed with either a meat or vegetarian filling, then braised; the vegetarian filling is given below. Served with a green vegetable and rice, this constitutes a rich and tasty main course.

Variation

For a vegetarian dish, replace the meat with 7 oz (210 g) finely diced eggplant. Mix eggplant with 1 tsp (5 mL) salt and let sit 20 minutes. Wrap eggplant in cloth or paper towels and squeeze out as much liquid as you can. Proceed with recipe as above, reducing added salt to 1/8 tsp (0.5 mL) and replacing chicken stock with vegetable stock.

2 lbs	bean curd or firm tofu, cut into 6 pieces, about 2 1/2 inches (7 cm) square	1 kg
1/4 cup	cornstarch	50 mL
1 cup	vegetable oil	250 mL
2 tbsp	finely chopped green onion, white part only	25 mL
6 oz	ground pork	175 g
1/4 tsp	white pepper	1 mL
1 cup	finely chopped mushrooms	250 mL
2 tsp	Chinese rice wine or dry sherry or sake	10 mL
1/4 tsp	salt	1 mL
1	beaten egg	1
2 tbsp	finely chopped green onion, green part only	25 mL
2 tbsp	finely chopped Chinese celery, coriander or parsley	25 mL
1 tbsp	cornstarch	15 mL
1/2 tsp	sesame oil	2 mL
2 tbsp	grated ginger root	25 mL
1 cup	chicken stock	250 mL
2 tbsp	soya sauce	25 mL

1. Drain and rinse bean curd; weigh down with a plate for at least 30 minutes to remove excess water. Pat dry with paper towels. Dip all sides in cornstarch, shaking off extra. In a nonstick frying pan, heat oil over medium-high heat; when oil is hot, cook bean curd for 5 minutes per side or until golden. Drain on paper towel. Cool.

2. Remove all but 1 tbsp (15 mL) oil from the frying pan; cook white part of green onion until softened. Stir in pork and pepper; cook, stirring, until no longer pink. Stir in mushrooms; cook for 30 seconds. Stir in rice wine and salt; cook until liquid evaporates. Remove from heat; cool. Drain off any liquid, adding it to the stock. Mix meat with egg, green part of green onion, celery, cornstarch and sesame oil.

3. Cut each cooked bean curd cake in half horizontally. Scoop 2 tsp (10 mL) of bean curd from center of each half; fill indentation in each bottom half with meat filling, mounding it up, and cover with a top half.

4. Wrap ginger in a piece of cheesecloth and squeeze out juice over a bowl. Mix ginger pulp with 2 tbsp (25 mL) of the stock and squeeze out juice through cheesecloth again. In a large shallow saucepan, combine ginger juice, remaining stock and soya sauce; bring to a simmer over medium heat. Carefully add stuffed bean curd cakes, cover and simmer for 12 minutes. Transfer cakes to warm serving platter; cut in half diagonally with a sharp knife. Bring sauce to a boil; cook until slightly thickened and pour over bean curd.

Braised roasted pork with tofu and green onions

Serves 4 to 6

Crispy-skinned and succulent roasted pork, sold by the pound, is one of our favorite treats from the Chinese barbecue shop. It's hard not to eat it right away, but if there's anything left, this is a great way to use it up.

4	dried Chinese black mushrooms	4
1 tbsp	vegetable oil	15 mL
5	thin slices ginger root	5
1 tsp	minced garlic	5 mL
1 lb	crispy-skin roasted pork or barbecued pork or leftover roast pork, cut into 1/2-inch (1 cm) slices	500 g
2 tbsp	oyster sauce	25 mL
1 tbsp	soya sauce	15 mL
1 tbsp	dark soya sauce	15 mL
1/2 cup	chicken stock *or* water	125 mL
	Salt and freshly ground black pepper to taste	
1 tbsp	cornstarch, dissolved in 2 tbsp (25 mL) chicken stock or water	15 mL
2	packages (10 oz [300 g]) soft tofu, cut into pieces 1 inch (2.5 cm) by 1/2 inch (1 cm)	2
3	green onions, cut into 1-inch (2.5 cm) lengths	3

1. In a heatproof bowl, soak mushrooms in boiling water for 15 minutes. Remove stems, slice caps thinly and set aside.

2. In a wok or deep skillet, heat oil over medium-high heat. Add ginger root, garlic and mushrooms and sauté until fragrant (about 1 minute). Add pork and stir-fry for 1 minute. Add oyster sauce, soya sauce, dark soya sauce and stock; mix well. Reduce heat to medium and cook for 3 minutes. Season to taste with salt and pepper. Add dissolved cornstarch and cook until sauce is thickened.

3. Gently fold tofu and green onions into mixture; cover and allow to absorb flavors for 2 minutes. Transfer to a deep platter and serve immediately.

Bistro lentils with smoked sausage

Serves 6

It's Friday night. You've worked hard all week. Don't even bother setting the table. Here's a supper dish that's easy to balance on your lap while you relax in front of the TV set. As an added bonus, this dish goes great with a cold beer.

Tip

Any kind of smoked sausage or ham works well. The smaller-sized green Laird lentils hold their shape in cooking and are the kind I prefer for this recipe.

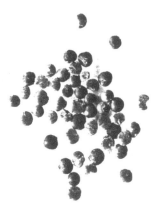

3 1/2 cups	chicken stock or vegetable stock (approximate)	875 mL
1 1/2 cups	lentils, picked over and rinsed	375 mL
1/2 tsp	dried thyme	2 mL
2 tbsp	olive oil	25 mL
1 cup	diced red onions	250 mL
3	cloves garlic, finely chopped	3
2	carrots, peeled and diced	2
1 cup	diced fennel or celery	250 mL
1	red bell pepper, diced	1
2 tbsp	balsamic vinegar	25 mL
8 oz	smoked sausage, such as kielbasa, cut into 1/2-inch (1 cm) chunks	250 g
	Black pepper	
1/4 cup	chopped fresh parsley	50 mL

1. In a large saucepan, bring stock to a boil over high heat; add lentils and thyme. Reduce heat to medium-low and simmer, covered, for 25 to 30 minutes or until lentils are just tender but still hold their shape.

2. Meanwhile, heat oil in a large nonstick skillet over medium heat. Add onions, garlic, carrots and fennel; cook, stirring often, for 8 minutes. Add red pepper; cook, stirring, for 2 minutes or until vegetables are just tender. Stir in vinegar; remove from heat.

3. Add vegetables and smoked sausage to lentils in saucepan; season to taste with pepper. Cover and cook for 5 to 8 minutes or until sausage is heated through. (Add more stock or water, if necessary, to prevent lentils from sticking.) Stir in parsley. Serve warm or at room temperature.

Serves 6

Involtini con fagioloni bianchi
Stuffed veal rolls with white beans

Make sure the veal you use here is as thin as possible. To achieve this, place veal slices between sheets of waxed paper and gently pound with a kitchen mallet or rolling pin, being careful not to tear the meat.

Sauce

1/4 cup	olive oil	50 mL
2 oz	pancetta, chopped	50 g
3	cloves garlic, finely chopped	3
1	medium onion, finely chopped	1
1/4 cup	finely chopped flat-leaf parsley	50 mL
4	large plum tomatoes, peeled and chopped or canned Italian plum tomatoes, drained	4
3 cups	cooked white beans	750 mL

Filling

8 oz	mushrooms, minced	250 g
1/3 cup	dry red wine	75 mL
4 oz	Italian salami, finely chopped	125 g
1/3 cup	grated Parmigiano-Reggiano	75 mL
1	egg	1
1/2 tsp	salt	2 mL
1/4 tsp	freshly ground black pepper	1 mL
	Dry bread crumbs, as needed	
2 lbs	veal (about 12 slices)	1 kg
1/4 cup	butter	50 mL

1. In a skillet, heat half of the olive oil over medium heat. Add pancetta, 2 of the chopped garlic cloves, the onion and half of the parsley; cook until onion is softened. Add tomatoes and beans; cook for 15 minutes or until slightly thickened. Season with salt and pepper to taste. Transfer beans/sauce mixture to a bowl; set aside.

2. Wipe the skillet clean and sauté remaining garlic in remaining olive oil. Add mushrooms and cook, stirring, for 1 minute. Add wine and cook until it is absorbed by mushrooms. Allow mushroom mixture to cool, then mix with the salami, Parmigiano-Reggiano, egg, salt and pepper. (Add a small amount of dry bread crumbs if too wet.)

3. Spread some of this mixture on each of the veal scallops. Roll slices up firmly and secure each with a toothpick. Wipe skillet clean.

4. Over medium heat, heat butter in the skillet; cook the veal rolls, turning once or twice, for 8 to 10 minutes or until golden brown. (Do not overcook, or they will toughen.) Add beans and their sauce and simmer gently for 15 minutes or until heated through. Serve immediately.

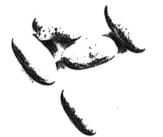

Lentils with saffron-scented meat

Serves 4

Bolstered with additional vegetables, this rib-sticking lentil stew is partnered with meat that is smoky and heady from saffron and garlic. It'll transform even the coldest winter night into an occasion of cozy comfort, especially if served alongside rice and greens. In keeping with our lean and mean modern tastes, precious little oil (in fact, the bare minimum) is called for here. Therefore, a drizzle of some fine olive oil (chili-spiced if you like) at table will add immeasurably to the appeal of these lentils.

13- BY 9-INCH (3 L) BAKING DISH
PREHEAT OVEN TO 400° F (200° C)

1 cup	green lentils, rinsed and drained	250 mL
4 1/2 cups	boiling water	1.125 L
1	carrot, scraped and finely diced (about 1/2 cup [125 mL])	1
1	potato, peeled and finely diced (about 1 cup [250 mL])	1
2 cups	finely diced onions (about 2 medium)	500 mL
1	stalk celery with leaves, finely chopped	1
1/4 cup	finely chopped garlic	50 mL
1 tsp	balsamic vinegar	5 mL
1/2 tsp	dried basil	2 mL
1/2 tsp	dried oregano	2 mL
1 tsp	granulated sugar	5 mL
1/4 tsp	freshly ground black pepper	1 mL
	Salt to taste	
1/4 cup	olive oil	50 mL
1/4 tsp	freshly ground black pepper	1 mL
1/2 tsp	saffron threads	2 mL
1 lb	ground pork or lamb or beef (or a combination)	500 g
	Salt to taste	
2	medium tomatoes, cut into 1/4-inch (5 mm) rounds (about 1 lb [500 g])	2
	Few sprigs fresh basil or parsley, chopped	
	Extra virgin olive oil	

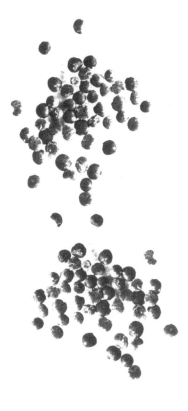

1. In a large pot, soak lentils in 2 cups (500 mL) of the boiling water for 20 minutes. (They will swell up and absorb most of the water.)

2. Add remaining 2 1/2 cups (625 mL) boiling water. Stir in carrot, potato, 1 cup (250 mL) of the onions, celery, 2 tbsp (25 mL) of the garlic, vinegar, basil, oregano, sugar and 1/4 tsp (1 mL) black pepper. Bring to a boil; reduce heat to medium and cook uncovered, stirring very occasionally, for 45 minutes. (It should have steady but not vigorous bubbles.) By now the lentils and vegetables should be tender but still holding their shape, and the water mostly absorbed. Season to taste with salt.

3. Meanwhile, in a large frying pan, heat olive oil with 1/4 tsp (1 mL) black pepper over high heat for 1 minute. Add remaining 1 cup (250 mL) onions; stir-fry for 2 minutes or until almost charring. Add remaining garlic and saffron; stir-fry for 30 seconds. Add ground meat; stir-fry, folding to break it up, for 2 to 3 minutes or until no longer pink. Reduce heat to medium-low, cover and cook 3 to 4 minutes or until meat is cooked through and flavorful. Remove from heat. Season to taste with salt; set aside.

4. Transfer cooked lentils to baking dish, spreading them evenly over bottom of dish. Spread the meat and its juices evenly over the lentils. Cover the entire surface of the meat with sliced tomatoes. Bake uncovered for 30 minutes or until the tomatoes have withered and the lentils are happily bubbling.

5. Remove from oven and let rest for 5 minutes. Serve large portions, garnished with chopped herbs, and a beaker of olive oil for drizzling at table.

Braised lamb with beans and dates

Serves 4 or 5

Choose a cold winter night and dazzle the loved ones with this sweet-hot stew and its soothing beans and carrots (ideal alongside rice). The sweetness comes from dates (pitted, please), while the heat from crushed chilies provides a necessary counterpoint to the ultimately cloying effect of a sweet-only sauce. If chilies absolutely don't agree with you (a real pity), substitute 1 tsp (5 mL) white wine vinegar (add along with the chicken stock) for a sweet-and-sour result.

2 tbsp	olive oil	25 mL
1/2 tsp	ground allspice	2 mL
1/2 tsp	ground cumin	2 mL
1/2 tsp	salt	2 mL
1/4 tsp	freshly ground black pepper	1 mL
2 cups	finely diced onions	500 mL
1/4 to 1/2 tsp	chili flakes, or to taste	1 to 2 mL
2 1/2 lbs	lamb leg or shoulder cut into 1 1/2-inch (4 cm) pieces (bone in, fat trimmed)	1.25 kg
1	large carrot, peeled and cut into 1/4-inch (5 mm) rounds	1
2	stalks celery with leaves, finely chopped	2
1 cup	diced peeled tomatoes, with juice or canned tomatoes	250 mL
3 cups	boiling chicken stock	750 mL
1 tsp	dried oregano	5 mL
1 tsp	dried thyme	5 mL
1 cup	pitted dates (about 4 oz [125 g])	250 mL
2 cups	cooked white kidney beans or 1 can (19 oz [540 mL]), rinsed and drained	500 mL
1/4 cup	packed chopped fresh parsley	50 mL
	Steamed rice as an accompaniment	

1. In a large saucepan, heat olive oil, allspice, cumin, salt and pepper over high heat, stirring, for 1 minute. Add onions and chili flakes; stir-fry for 4 minutes or until starting to brown. Add lamb and cook, stirring actively, for 5 to 7 minutes or until the lamb is thoroughly browned and everything is well mixed together. Add carrot, celery, tomatoes, chicken stock, oregano and thyme; mix together to settle everything in the liquid.

2. Bring to a boil and reduce heat to medium. Cook uncovered for 45 minutes or until the lamb is tender. Stir every 15 minutes and keep up a steady but not vigorous bubble.

3. Fold in dates, beans and parsley; wait for the steady-but-not-vigorous bubble to return. Cook for 20 minutes, folding from the bottom up every 5 minutes to avoid scorching. Remove from heat and cover. Let rest for 5 to 10 minutes.

4. Portion alongside steamed rice with plenty of sauce; serve immediately.

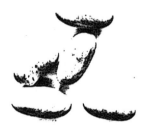

Serves 6

Stinco d'agnello con purée di fave
Lamb shanks with fava bean purée

Chef Massimo Capra of Mistura tells me that in Apulia, the fava bean purée and chicory included here would be served first on their own, followed by the lamb and its sauce teamed with boiled potatoes. However you choose to serve it, this is one outstanding preparation.

Plan to make the bean purée the day before.

To save time and effort, buy skinned, dried fava beans. Simply rinse, cover with cold water and bring to a boil; turn heat off and let stand 1 hour. Purée and proceed with recipe as described in step 3.

3 tbsp	olive oil	45 mL
6	lamb shanks	6
2	carrots, scraped and chopped	2
2	onions, chopped	2
3	stalks celery, chopped	3
4	bay leaves	4
5	branches rosemary	5
	Salt and freshly ground black pepper to taste	
1 1/2 cups	dry white wine	375 mL
6 cups	chicken stock	1.5 L
1 lb	whole dried fava beans, soaked overnight and drained	500 g
3	cloves garlic, finely chopped	3
1/2 tsp	salt	2 mL
1/4 cup	olive oil	50 mL
2 tbsp	butter	25 mL
3 tbsp	extra virgin olive oil	45 mL
1 lb	broccoli rabe (or other bitter greens such as dandelion, turnip or collard greens), chopped and blanched	500 g

1. In a casserole or Dutch oven, heat olive oil over high heat. Add lamb shanks and sear until golden brown. Add carrots, onions, celery, bay leaves, rosemary, salt and pepper; continue cooking for a few minutes. Add wine and cook for 5 minutes to allow alcohol to evaporate. Add half of the stock and simmer, covered, for 1 1/2 hours over very low heat.

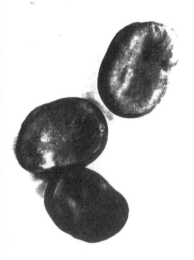

2. Meanwhile, make the fava purée: Pull outer skin off each fava bean. Place peeled beans and garlic in a saucepan; add fresh water to cover and cook for 1 hour or until tender, skimming off any foam that rises to the surface. When foam stops appearing, add salt; stir beans occasionally with a wooden spoon to help them break up. Keep some water boiling to add to the beans as they cook to keep them from sticking to the bottom of the pan.

3. Once the beans are completely cooked, mash them to a purée with 1/4 cup (50 mL) olive oil. (Alternatively, put them through a food mill or into a food processor and blend with olive oil until smooth.) Season to taste.

4. When meat is tender, carefully remove it to a warm serving platter; cover and set to one side. Keep lamb warm. Bring liquid to a boil and cook until reduced by one-third (about 1 hour). Add butter and season to taste. Strain liquid through a fine sieve into a small saucepan; keep warm.

5. In a skillet heat the remaining olive oil over medium heat. Add the chopped, blanched greens and a little salt and pepper; sauté until slightly wilted.

6. To serve, place one scoop of bean purée and greens in the center of a rimmed pasta plate. Top with one lamb shank and pour the juices around the vegetables. Serve immediately.

Chuckwagon beef shortribs and beans

Serves 8 to 10

Cluny-area rancher Leo Maynard gave me this recipe — the winner of a bean contest I once organized. (But then, how could he not win after he pulled into the newspaper parking lot with his chuckwagon and set up a wood stove to cook this tasty combination of Alberta beef and beans?) Leo also gave me my first taste of real prairie oysters, roasted over a campfire at a cowboy cooking contest — and another of my very favorite things, my orange kitty, O.J.

Leo serves this excellent chili with his own homemade biscuits.

If dried pinto beans are unavailable, use Romano or red kidney beans.

After browning ribs and cooking onions on the stove top, you can also put everything in a slow cooker and cook for 6 to 8 hours.

2 tbsp	canola oil	25 mL
4 lbs	beef short ribs, cut into pieces	2 kg
4	chopped onions	4
1 lb	dried pinto beans (about 3 cups [750 mL]) soaked overnight in water to cover)	500 g
1	can (8 oz [213 mL]) tomato sauce	1
1/2 cup	packed brown sugar	125 mL
2 tbsp	prepared mustard	25 mL
2 tbsp	chili powder	25 mL
1 tbsp	cider vinegar	15 mL
2 tsp	liquid smoke	10 mL
1 tsp	Worcestershire sauce	5 mL
2 tsp	salt	10 mL

1. In a large Dutch oven, heat oil over medium-high heat; in several batches, cook rib pieces, turning occasionally, for 5 minutes or until browned on all sides. With a slotted spoon, transfer ribs to a bowl leaving behind as much oil as possible. Reduce heat to medium; add onions and cook, stirring occasionally, for 8 minutes or until tender.

2. Stir in 6 cups (1.5 L) water, drained beans, tomato sauce, brown sugar, mustard, chili powder, vinegar, liquid smoke, Worcestershire sauce and half of the salt; bring to a boil. Place browned ribs on top. Reduce heat to low and simmer, covered, for 5 hours or until beans and ribs are tender. Season to taste with remaining salt.

Chicken fagioli
Bean tomato sauce

Serves 4

Tip
Use bone-in chicken breasts instead of legs; reduce browning time to 4 minutes and reduce cooking time to 20 minutes.

White kidney beans or a combination can be used.

A great dish to reheat.

Make Ahead
Brown chicken earlier in the day and refrigerate until ready to cook with sauce.

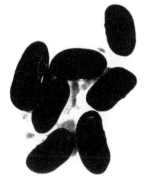

2 tsp	vegetable oil	10 mL
4	chicken legs	4
1/4 cup	all-purpose flour	50 mL
2 tsp	minced garlic	10 mL
1/2 cup	chopped onions	125 mL
1/3 cup	chopped carrots	75 mL
1/3 cup	chopped celery	75 mL
1 1/2 cups	red kidney beans, drained	375 mL
1 cup	puréed canned tomatoes	250 mL
3/4 cup	chicken stock	175 mL
1 1/2 tsp	dried basil	7 mL
1 tsp	dried oregano	5 mL

1. In a large nonstick skillet sprayed with vegetable spray, heat 1 tsp (5 mL) of the oil over high heat. Dust chicken with flour and cook, turning often, for 8 minutes or until browned on all sides. Set aside and wipe skillet clean.

2. Reduce heat to medium. Add remaining 1 tsp (5 mL) oil to skillet. Add garlic, onions, carrots and celery; cook for 5 minutes or until softened. Mash 1/2 cup (125 mL) of the kidney beans; add mashed and whole beans, tomatoes, stock, basil and oregano to skillet. Bring to a boil; reduce heat to medium-low. Add browned chicken pieces and cook, covered, for 30 minutes or until juices run clear when legs are pierced at thickest point. Stir occasionally. Remove skin before eating.

Chicken tortillas

Serves 4

Tip
Boneless turkey breast, pork or veal scallopini can replace chicken.

The cheese adds a creamy texture to the tortillas. Mozzarella can also be used.

Make Ahead
Prepare filling early in the day and gently reheat before stuffing tortillas. Add extra stock if sauce is too thick.

PREHEAT OVEN TO 375° F (190° C)
BAKING SHEET SPRAYED WITH VEGETABLE SPRAY

6 oz	skinless boneless chicken breast, diced	150 g
1 tsp	vegetable oil	5 mL
1 tsp	crushed garlic	5 mL
1 cup	chopped onions	250 mL
1/2 cup	finely chopped carrots	125 mL
1 cup	tomato pasta sauce	250 mL
1 cup	canned red kidney beans, drained	250 mL
1/2 cup	chicken stock	125 mL
1 tsp	chili powder	5 mL
8	small 6-inch (15 cm) flour tortillas	8
1/2 cup	shredded Cheddar cheese (optional)	125 mL

1. In a nonstick skillet sprayed with vegetable spray, cook chicken over high heat for 2 minutes or until done at center. Remove from skillet and set aside.

2. Reduce heat to medium and add oil to pan. Respray with vegetable spray and cook garlic, onions, and carrots for 10 minutes or until browned and softened, stirring often. Add some water if vegetables start to burn. Add tomato sauce, beans, stock and chili powder and cook for 10 to 12 minutes or until carrots are tender, mixture has thickened and most of the liquid is absorbed. Stir in chicken and remove from heat.

3. Put 1/3 cup (75 mL) mixture on each tortilla; sprinkle with cheese (if using) and roll up. Put on prepared baking sheet and bake in preheated oven for 10 minutes or until heated through.

Serves 6

A thoroughly enjoyable combination favored by Chef Massimo Capra – and by me too! "People don't think of putting beans and shrimp together but it is very traditional and delicious," says the chef. A lovely addition to an antipasto spread, it also makes a wonderfully light first course. Serve with good crusty Italian bread to mop up the rich juices.

It is important that the beans are hot when combined with the other ingredients so they will absorb all the flavors.

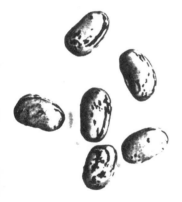

Gamberi e fagioli alla Massimo
Massimo's shrimp and beans

1 lb	dried romano beans, soaked overnight in water to cover	500 g
1	large red onion, thinly sliced	1
3	cloves garlic, minced	3
3/4 cup	lemon juice	175 mL
1/4 cup	extra virgin olive oil	50 mL
	Salt and freshly ground black pepper	
6 tbsp	butter	90 mL
2 lbs	medium shrimp (fresh or thawed from frozen), peeled and deveined	1 kg
3	large ripe plum tomatoes, diced	3
1 cup	chopped flat-leaf parsley	250 mL
1	bunch frisée or other salad greens, washed and trimmed	1

1. In a large saucepan, combine drained beans with cold water to cover by 2 inches (5 cm). Bring to a boil, reduce heat to simmer and cook 1 1/2 hours or until beans are tender. Drain.

2. In a bowl stir together hot beans, red onion, half the garlic, half the lemon juice and olive oil. Season to taste with salt and pepper. Cover with plastic wrap and keep in a warm place.

3. In a large skillet, melt butter over medium-high heat. Add shrimp, remaining garlic and remaining lemon juice; cook, stirring often, for 5 minutes or until shrimp are pink. Season to taste with salt and pepper.

4. Stir tomatoes and parsley into warm bean mixture. Pour onto a large serving platter; top with shrimp and their pan juices. Arrange frisée around edges and serve immediately.

Serves 4

This is one of our favorite adaptations from classical Cantonese cooking.

If you've been telling yourself to eat more tofu for its health benefits, this should convince you that it can also be delicious.

Steamed shrimp-stuffed tofu with broccoli

PREHEAT STEAMER OVER MEDIUM-HIGH HEAT

Stuffing

8 oz	raw shrimp, coarsely chopped	250 g
1 tsp	minced ginger root	5 mL
1/2 cup	water chestnuts, finely chopped	125 mL
2 tbsp	finely chopped green onions	25 mL
1	egg white, beaten	1
1/4 tsp	salt	1 mL
1 tbsp	cornstarch	15 mL
1 lb	soft tofu	500 g
2 cups	broccoli florets, cut into bite-sized pieces	500 mL

Sauce

2 tsp	sesame oil	10 mL
2 tbsp	soya sauce	25 mL
1 tbsp	chicken stock	15 mL
Pinch	granulated sugar	Pinch

1. In a mixing bowl, combine shrimp, ginger root, water chestnuts, green onions, egg white, salt and cornstarch; mix well and set aside.

2. Drain liquid from tofu package. Gently cut tofu in half lengthwise, then slice each half into 1/2-inch (1 cm) thick slices. Gently pat pieces dry with paper towel. Lay tofu pieces in a flat layer in the center of a plate that will fit into steamer. Line the outside of the plate with a ring of broccoli florets. Spoon a portion (about 1 tbsp [15 mL]) of shrimp stuffing onto each slice of tofu, pressing gently with the back of the spoon so it sticks to the tofu.

3. Place the plate in preheated steamer, cover and steam for 5 minutes or until shrimp mixture is firm to the touch.

4. In a small saucepan over medium-high heat, combine sesame oil, soya sauce, stock and sugar; heat just until boiling. Pour sauce evenly over cooked tofu and broccoli; serve immediately.

Serves 4

Salmon over white-and-black bean salsa

Swordfish or tuna can be substituted for salmon.

Other varieties of beans can be substituted if black or white navy beans are unavailable.

If you're not using canned beans, 1 cup (250 mL) dry yields 3 cups (750 mL) cooked.

Make Ahead
Prepare bean mixture earlier in the day and keep refrigerated. Stir before serving.

START BARBECUE OR PREHEAT OVEN TO 425° F (220° C)

1 cup	canned black beans, drained	250 mL
1 cup	canned white navy beans, drained	250 mL
3/4 cup	chopped tomatoes	175 mL
1/2 cup	chopped green bell peppers	125 mL
1/4 cup	chopped red onions	50 mL
1/4 cup	chopped fresh coriander	50 mL
2 tbsp	balsamic vinegar	25 mL
2 tbsp	lemon juice	25 mL
1 tbsp	olive oil	15 mL
1 tsp	minced garlic	5 mL
1 lb	salmon steaks	500 g

1. In a bowl combine black beans, white beans, tomatoes, green peppers, red onions and coriander. In a small bowl, whisk together vinegar, lemon juice, olive oil and garlic; pour over bean mixture and toss to combine.

2. Barbecue salmon or bake uncovered for approximately 10 minutes per 1-inch (2.5 cm) thickness or until fish flakes with a fork. Serve over bean salsa.

Pasta and Grains

Linguine with tuna, white beans and dill

Serves 6

Tip

For color variation, try red kidney beans or black beans instead of white beans.

For a more sophisticated meal, replace canned tuna with cooked tuna or sword-fish.

Make Ahead

Prepare sauce up to a day ahead. Reheat gently, adding more stock if too thick.

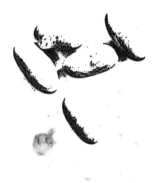

12 oz	linguine	375 g
1 tbsp	olive oil	15 mL
2 tsp	crushed garlic	10 mL
1	can (19 oz [540 mL]) white kidney beans, drained	1
4 tbsp	lemon juice	60 mL
1 3/4 cups	cold chicken stock	425 mL
4 tsp	all-purpose flour	20 mL
1	can (6.5 oz [185 g]) flaked tuna packed in water, drained	1
1/2 cup	chopped fresh dill (or 1 tbsp [15 mL] dried)	125 mL
1/3 cup	sliced black olives	75 mL
1/4 cup	chopped green onions	50 mL

1. Cook pasta in boiling water according to package instructions or until firm to the bite. Drain and place in a serving bowl.

2. In a large nonstick skillet, heat oil; add garlic, beans and lemon juice. Cook for 2 minutes or until hot.

3. Meanwhile, in a small bowl combine stock and flour until smooth. Add to bean mixture; simmer for 3 minutes or until sauce thickens slightly. Pour over pasta. Add tuna, dill, olives and green onions. Toss to combine.

Manicotti stuffed with chickpeas and cheese

Serves 4 to 5

PREHEAT OVEN TO 350° F (180° C)

9- BY 13-INCH BAKING DISH (3 L) SPRAYED WITH VEGETABLE SPRAY

10	manicotti shells	10
Sauce		
2 tsp	margarine *or* butter	10 mL
1 tbsp	all-purpose flour	15 mL
1/2 cup	2% milk	125 mL
1/2 cup	chicken stock	125 mL
2 tbsp	grated Parmesan cheese	25 mL
1 1/2 cups	canned chickpeas, drained	375 mL
1 cup	5% ricotta cheese	250 mL
1/2 cup	chopped green onions (about 4 medium)	125 mL
1/3 cup	grated Cheddar cheese	75 mL
1	egg	1
2 tbsp	grated Parmesan cheese	25 mL
1 1/2 tsp	minced garlic	7 mL
1 tsp	dried basil	5 mL
1 tbsp	grated Parmesan cheese	15 mL

1. In a large pot of boiling water, cook pasta according to package directions or until tender but firm; rinse under cold water and drain.

2. In a saucepan, melt margarine over medium heat; add flour and cook, stirring, for 1 minute. Gradually add milk and stock; stir constantly for 7 minutes or until sauce begins to simmer and thicken slightly. Stir in Parmesan and remove from heat.

3. Put chickpeas, ricotta, green onions, Cheddar cheese, egg, Parmesan, garlic and basil in food processor; pulse on and off until well mixed. Stuff 3 tbsp (45 mL) into each shell and put in prepared dish. Pour white sauce over and sprinkle with remaining Parmesan. Bake, covered, for 15 minutes or until heated through.

Rice and red lentil pilaf with fried zucchini

Serves 4

Most "modern" types of cuisine borrow from a number of cultures to create a brand new dish. And this aromatic rice-and-red-lentil concoction is a perfect example. It could have come from India just as easily as from Turkey, while its fried zucchini garnish is strictly Greek. It entails several different procedures but they're all easy and can be performed at leisure — one by one, not simultaneously. The result is satisfyingly exotic and tasty, a most viable (and healthier) alternative to pasta for a light supper or lunch.

1/2 cup	red lentils (*masoor dal*)	125 mL
1 cup	water	250 mL
1/2 tsp	salt	2 mL
1/4 cup	olive oil	50 mL
1/4 tsp	ground cinnamon	1 mL
1/4 tsp	ground cumin	1 mL
1/4 tsp	turmeric	1 mL
1/2 tsp	salt	2 mL
1/4 tsp	freshly ground black pepper	1 mL
3/4 cup	finely diced onions	175 mL
1/2 cup	finely diced red bell peppers	125 mL
2 tbsp	finely chopped garlic	25 mL
2 tbsp	dried currants	25 mL
1/2 cup	short-grain rice	125 mL
2 cups	boiling chicken stock	500 mL
1	zucchini (about 8 oz [250 g])	1
3 tbsp	all-purpose flour	45 mL
Pinch	salt	Pinch

1. Rinse and drain lentils. Put in a saucepan with water and 1/2 tsp (2 mL) salt. Bring to a boil. Remove from heat; pour into a bowl. Let soak for 10 to 15 minutes (the lentils will absorb most of the water).

2. Meanwhile in a heavy-bottomed pot with a tight-fitting lid over high heat, combine 2 tbsp (25 mL) of the oil, cinnamon, cumin, turmeric, salt and pepper. Cook, stirring, for 1 minute. Add onions and red peppers; stir-fry for 2 minutes or until beginning to char. Add garlic and currants; stir-fry for 1 minute.

(Recipe continues...)

CHICKPEA TOFU STEW (PAGE 100) ➤
OVERLEAF, LEFT: BEAN AND SWEET POTATO CHILI ON GARLIC POLENTA (PAGE 103)
OVERLEAF, RIGHT: SPINACH DAL (PAGE 168)

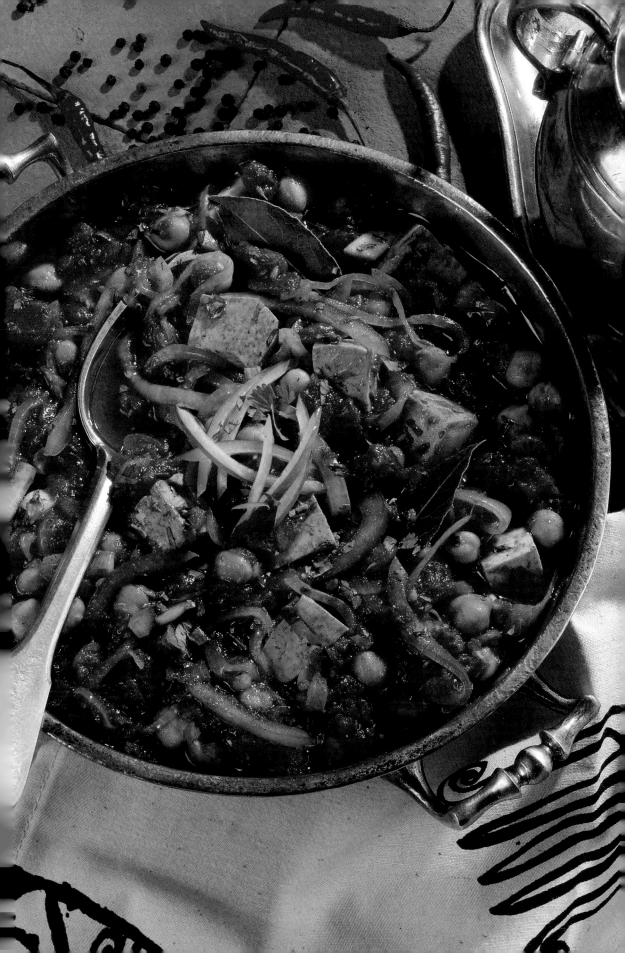

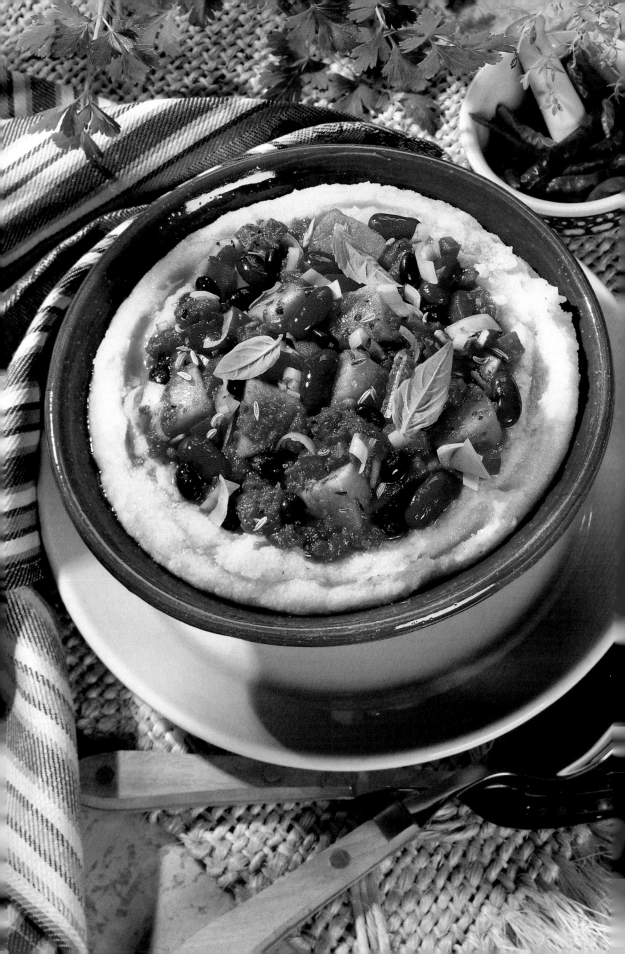

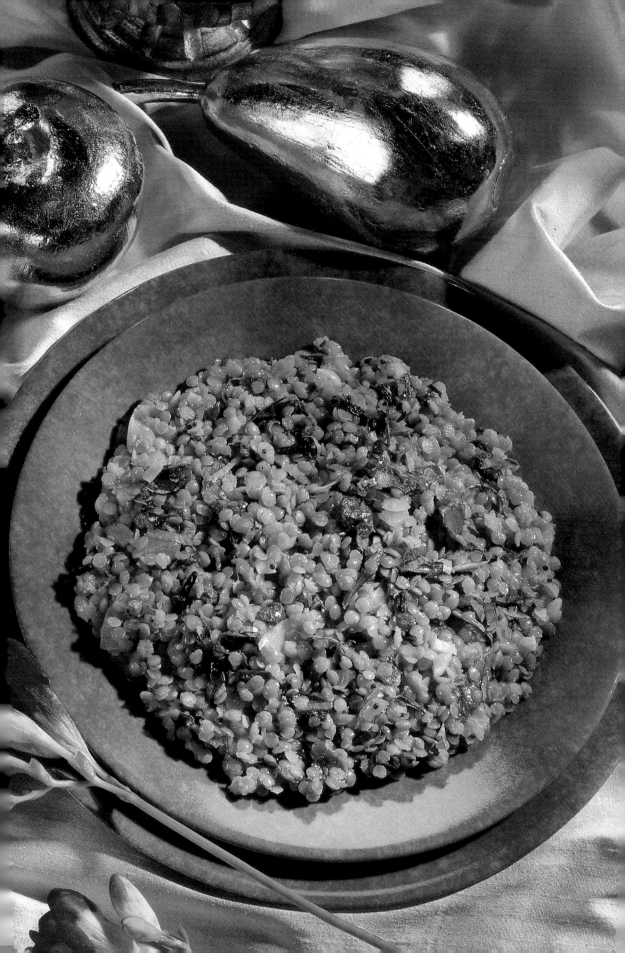

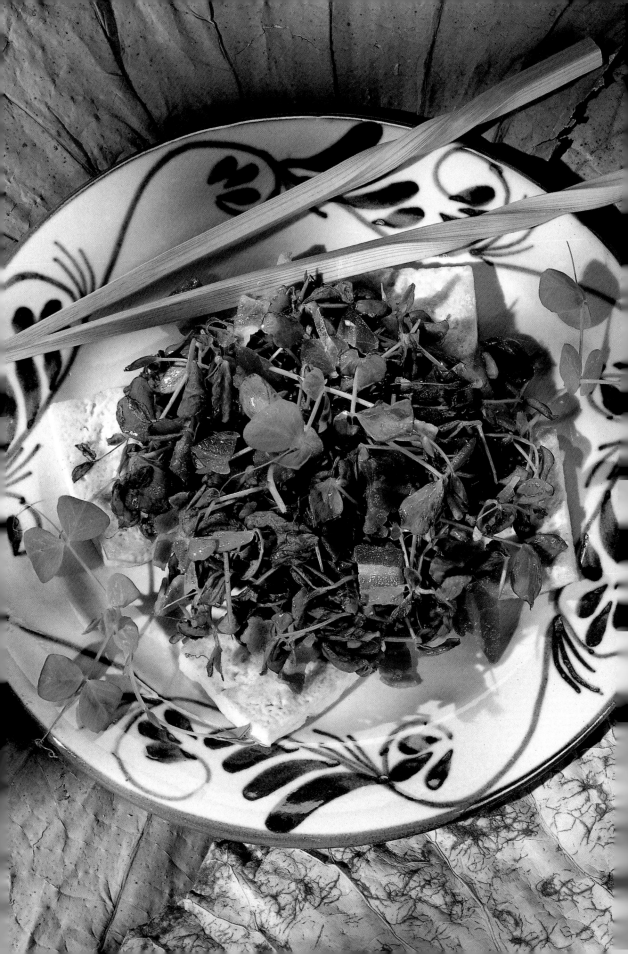

3. Immediately drain the leftover water from the lentils; add to pot along with rice. Cook, stirring, for 1 minute or until rice and lentils are coated with oil. Add chicken stock and stir to settle everything evenly in the liquid. Reduce heat to low and cover the pot tightly. Cook undisturbed for 20 minutes. Remove from heat. Let rest, covered, for 10 minutes.

4. Meanwhile, cut the zucchini lengthwise into long, thin (1/8- to 1/4-inch [3 to 5 mm]) slices (you should get 8 slices). Dredge lightly in flour. In a large frying pan, heat 2 tbsp (25 mL) olive oil and pinch of salt over high heat for 1 minute. Add zucchini in a single layer and fry each side for 2 minutes or until golden brown. Transfer to a paper towel-lined plate to drain excess oil.

5. Uncover rice/lentil mixture. Fluff, folding from the bottom up to distribute all ingredients throughout. Put portions onto 4 plates. Garnish with 2 slices of fried zucchini per portion and serve immediately.

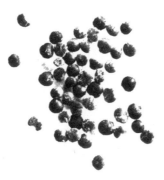

◄ Pea Tops with Pancetta and Tofu (Page 172)

Rice and black bean stuffed peppers

Serves 6

The Greeks stuff just about any vegetable they can get their hands on — from cabbage and vine leaves to zucchinis, tomatoes and eggplants. But peppers are their favorites, especially at harvest time, when they are so affordable. This is an heirloom recipe, which has been fleshed out with the addition of black beans, both for color and taste. These peppers are meant to be eaten at room temperature, when their various flavors really come to the fore. They make a perfect buffet item, especially because they can be (carefully) cut in half to double the number of servings. They also keep well (covered) in the fridge; just let them come back to room temperature before serving.

LARGE ROASTING PAN OR BAKING DISH
PREHEAT OVEN TO 375° F (190° C)

12	bell peppers, various colors	12
2 lbs	onions, stemmed and peeled	1 kg
1/2 tsp	ground cinnamon	2 mL
1/2 tsp	salt	2 mL
1/4 tsp	freshly ground black pepper	1 mL
1/4 cup	pine nuts	50 mL
1/4 cup	currants	50 mL
1/4 cup	olive oil	50 mL
1 cup	short-grain rice	250 mL
1 cup	diced peeled tomatoes, with juices *or* canned tomatoes	250 mL
1 1/2 cups	boiling water	375 mL
1/4 cup	chopped fresh mint (or 1 tbsp [15 mL] dried)	50 mL
1/4 cup	chopped fresh drill (or 1 tbsp [15 mL] dried)	50 mL
2 cups	cooked black beans *or* 1 can (19 oz [540 mL]) black beans, rinsed and drained	500 mL

1. Slice a 1/2-inch (1 cm) round (including the stem, if any) from the top of each pepper. Set these aside. (They'll serve later as "lids" for the stuffed peppers.) Trim the cavity of the peppers, discarding seed pod and seeds, without puncturing the walls or bottom of the peppers. Set aside.

2. In a bowl, shred the onions through the grater's largest holes (you'll have about 3 cups [750 mL] grated onions and juices). Transfer to a large nonstick frying pan. Add cinnamon, salt and pepper; cook, stirring, over high heat for 5 minutes or until most of the juices have evaporated. Add pine nuts, currants and olive oil; cook, stirring, for 3 minutes or until the onions start to catch on bottom of pan.

3. Immediately add rice; cook, stirring, for 2 minutes or until the rice is thoroughly coated with oil. Add tomatoes and 1/2 cup (125 mL) of the boiling water; cook, stirring, for about 4 minutes or until the tomatoes have broken down and the water is absorbed. Remove from heat. Stir in mint, dill and black beans until well mixed.

4. Stuff a scant 1/2 cup (125 mL) of the rice-bean stuffing into each pepper. (It should be about two-thirds full to allow for expansion.) Place stuffed peppers into roasting pan, fitting the peppers snugly in a single layer. Place the reserved tops on the peppers to act as lids. Add 1 cup (250 mL) boiling water around the peppers.

5. Cover and bake for 40 minutes, undisturbed. Uncover and bake for 30 to 40 minutes more to char the peppers and reduce the liquid. Remove from oven and cover the peppers. Let them cool down completely (about 1 1/2 hours) before serving.

Grilled polenta with sausage and chickpeas

Serves 4

Grits, mumaliga, cornmeal — whatever you call this stuff, it's a highly nutritious and versatile pudding made with milled corn and water. It can be enhanced with anything that strikes your fancy. Here it is broiled with a tiny brushing of olive oil and served on top of a savory sausage and chickpea stew. This dish is easy to make, inexpensive and impressive all at once.

Try it, even if you're put off by the notion of consuming anything that can be described as a "pudding." You'll come back to its comforts often, especially in the cold months.

PREHEAT BROILER
BAKING SHEET

2 1/2 cups	water	625 mL
1/2 tsp	salt	2 mL
1 cup	yellow cornmeal	250 mL
1 lb	Italian sausages (spicy or mild)	500 g
1	onion, sliced	1
Half	green bell pepper, sliced	Half
1 tbsp	olive oil	15 mL
1 tbsp	finely chopped garlic	15 mL
1/2 tsp	fennel seeds	2 mL
1 cup	finely chopped peeled tomatoes, with juices *or* canned tomatoes	250 mL
1 cup	white wine	250 mL
1 tsp	dried basil	5 mL
2 cups	cooked chickpeas *or* 1 can (19 oz [540 mL]) chickpeas, rinsed and drained	500 mL
6	black olives, pitted and quartered	6
1 tbsp	olive oil	15 mL
	Grated Romano cheese	
	Few sprigs fresh basil or parsley, chopped	

1. In a large deep saucepan, bring water to a rolling boil. Add salt. Reduce heat to low. Add cornmeal in a thin but steady stream, stirring constantly (preferably with a wooden spoon). Cook, stirring, for 2 to 3 minutes or until the mixture is smooth and has thickened to the consistency of mashed potatoes. Transfer the polenta to a medium-sized bowl and cover with an inverted plate. Let rest at least 10 minutes.

2. Meanwhile, broil sausages, onion and green pepper under a hot broiler for 3 to 4 minutes per side. The sausages should not cook through (neither should the onions and peppers burn). Take them out and slice the sausages into 1/2-inch (1 cm) pieces. Mix the sausages, onions and green peppers together; set aside.

3. In a deep frying pan, heat 1 tbsp (15 mL) olive oil over high heat for 30 seconds. Add garlic and fennel seeds; stir-fry for 1 minute or until sizzling. Add sausage, onions and peppers; stir-fry for 1 minute, turning the sausages to sear both sides of the slices. Add tomatoes and stir-fry for 2 minutes to break them up somewhat. Add wine and basil; cook, stirring, for 1 to 2 minutes or until everything is bubbling. Stir in chickpeas and olives. Reduce heat to medium-low, cover and cook for 15 minutes, undisturbed. Remove from heat. Stir, cover and let rest for 5 to 10 minutes to develop flavor.

4. Meanwhile, turn cooled polenta onto plate by inverting the bowl and giving it a tap. Cut the polenta into 1/2-inch (1 cm) slices (you should get about 12 slices). Brush baking sheet with 1 tbsp (15 mL) olive oil. Roll each polenta slice in oil on sheet to cover both sides. Arrange slices in a single layer on sheet. Broil polenta slices, without turning, for 6 to 7 minutes or until crusted and the edges are slightly charred.

5. Divide the stew between 4 plates. Top each with 3 slices of the grilled polenta. Sprinkle with cheese and garnish with basil. Serve immediately.

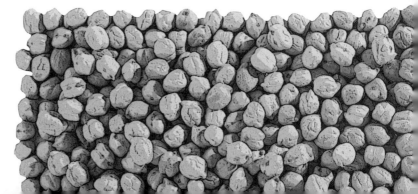

All-in-one pasta and chickpea ragout

Serves 4

You only need one pot to prepare this dish. Even the dried pasta is added to the very same pot and cooked until tender in the vegetable-tomato sauce. Spoon into bowls and sprinkle with shredded Fontina or Parmesan cheese.

Tip

Keep single servings on hand in the freezer for quick microwave meals.

Add 8 oz (250 g) cubed or sliced smoked sausage such as kielbasa or ham along with chickpeas.

1 tbsp	olive oil	15 mL
1	medium onion, chopped	1
2	cloves garlic, minced	2
1	large green bell pepper, chopped	1
1 tsp	dried oregano	5 mL
1/2 tsp	dried basil	2 mL
1/2 tsp	salt	2 mL
1/4 tsp	red pepper flakes	1 mL
1	can (28 oz [796 mL]) tomatoes, chopped	1
1 cup	vegetable stock	250 mL
1 cup	elbow macaroni	250 mL
2	small zucchini, halved length-wise and sliced	2
1	can (19 oz [540 mL]) chickpeas, rinsed and drained	1

1. In a Dutch oven or large saucepan, heat oil over medium heat. Add onion, garlic, pepper, oregano, basil, salt and red pepper flakes; cook, stirring, for 3 minutes or until vegetables are softened.

2. Add tomatoes and stock; bring to a boil. Reduce heat, cover and simmer, stirring occasionally, for 10 minutes. Stir in pasta; cover and cook for 5 minutes. Stir in zucchini and chickpeas; simmer for 5 to 7 minutes more or until pasta and zucchini are tender.

Penne with creamy white bean sauce

12 oz	penne	375 g
1	can (19 oz [540 mL]) white kidney beans, rinsed and drained	1
1 cup	vegetable stock, heated	250 mL
2 tbsp	olive oil	25 mL
2 tbsp	light mayonnaise	25 mL
1 tbsp	freshly squeezed lemon juice	15 mL
1 tbsp	drained capers	15 mL
1 1/2 tsp	minced garlic	7 mL
1/3 cup	chopped fresh dill (or 1 tbsp [15 mL] dried)	75 mL
1/4 tsp	freshly ground black pepper	1 mL
2 tsp	vegetable oil	10 mL
1 cup	chopped onions	250 mL
1 cup	chopped red bell peppers	250 mL
1 cup	fresh or frozen peas	250 mL

1. In a large pot of boiling water, cook penne for 8 to 10 minutes or until tender but firm. Meanwhile, prepare the sauce.

2. In a food processor, combine beans, stock, olive oil, mayonnaise, lemon juice, capers, garlic, dill and pepper; process until well mixed.

3. In a nonstick frying pan, heat oil over medium-high heat. Add onions and red peppers; cook 4 minutes or until browned. Stir in peas; cook for 1 minute.

4. Toss drained pasta with bean mixture and vegetables. Serve immediately.

Tip
Use any medium-sized pasta, such as rotini or medium shells.

Puréed kidney beans give this sauce a texture similar to canned tuna.

Add other vegetables to replace red peppers and peas. Snow peas, broccoli or sliced green beans are good choices.

Make Ahead
Prepare sauce early in the day. Sauté vegetables and cook pasta just before serving.

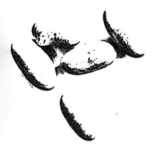

Curried couscous with tomatoes and chickpeas

Serves 4 to 6

2 cups	vegetable stock	500 mL
1 1/2 cups	couscous	375 mL
1 tsp	vegetable oil	5 mL
3 cups	chopped plum tomatoes	750 mL
1/2 cup	vegetable stock	125 mL
2 tsp	curry powder	10 mL
2 tsp	minced garlic	10 mL
2 cups	canned chickpeas, rinsed and drained	500 mL
3/4 cup	chopped fresh coriander	175 mL
1/2 cup	chopped green onions	125 mL

1. In a saucepan bring stock to a boil; stir in couscous, cover and remove from heat. Let stand 5 minutes; transfer to a serving bowl.
2. Meanwhile, in a large nonstick saucepan, heat oil over medium-high heat. Add tomatoes, stock, curry and garlic; cook, stirring, for 5 minutes or until tomatoes begin to break up. Stir in chickpeas; cook for 2 minutes or until heated through. Add to couscous along with coriander and green onions; toss to combine. Serve immediately.

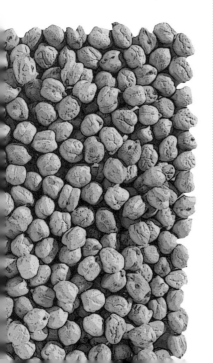

Hoisin stir-fried vegetables and tofu over rice noodles

Serves 4

Tip
Tofu is sold in the produce section of supermarkets. Be sure to use a firm or extra-firm variety or it will fall apart in the stir-fry.

Tofu can be replaced with 6 oz (175 g) cooked beans of your choice.

If rice noodles are unavailable, use regular pasta. Cook according to package directions.

Make Ahead
Prepare sauce up to 2 days in advance. Stir-fry just before serving.

Sauce

1/3 cup	hoisin sauce	75 mL
1/3 cup	soya sauce	75 mL
1/4 cup	rice wine vinegar	50 mL
1/4 cup	packed brown sugar	50 mL
1 tsp	minced garlic	5 mL
1 tsp	minced ginger root	5 mL

Stir-Fry

8 oz	thin rice vermicelli	250 g
2 tsp	vegetable oil	10 mL
2 1/4 cups	chopped red bell peppers	550 mL
2 1/4 cups	chopped leeks	550 mL
2 cups	sliced mushrooms	500 mL
1 1/4 cups	shredded carrots	300 mL
1 1/4 cups	chopped zucchini	300 mL
6 oz	firm tofu, cubed	175 g

1. In a small bowl, whisk together hoisin sauce, soya sauce, vinegar, brown sugar, garlic and ginger. Set aside.
2. Pour boiling water over noodles to cover; soak for 10 minutes or until soft. Drain well.
3. In a nonstick wok or large saucepan sprayed with vegetable spray, heat oil over high heat. Add red peppers and leeks; stir-fry for 4 minutes. Add mushrooms and stir-fry 2 minutes. Add carrots and zucchini; stir-fry 2 minutes or until vegetables are tender-crisp. Add noodles, tofu and sauce; stir-fry for 2 minutes or until bubbly and hot. Serve immediately.

Baked orzo and beans

Serves 4 to 6

Orzo — a jumbo rice looka-like — may be the most versatile of all pastas. This recipe comes from a long line of similarly baked Greek dishes, but borrows from Italian cuisine in its cheese topping. Use a plainer tomato sauce (mine may be too piquant) and omit the sautéed red onion, and you'll have a dish that delights young children, who seem to have a natural affinity to orzo (maybe because it's so much fun to pick up individual grains with tiny fingers).

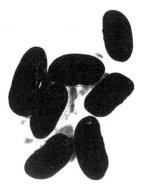

PREHEAT OVEN TO 350° F (180° C)
10-CUP (2.5 L) CASSEROLE WITH LID

2 1/2 cups	orzo	625 mL
1 tbsp	olive oil	15 mL
1/2 cup	sliced red onions	125 mL
2	tomatoes, roughly chopped	2
2 cups	tomato sauce	500 mL
2 cups	cooked red kidney beans	500 mL
1 cup	tomato juice	250 mL
1 cup	shaved Parmesan cheese	250 mL
1 tbsp	extra virgin olive oil	15 mL
	Few sprigs fresh parsley, chopped	
	Grated Romano (optional)	

1. In a large pot of boiling salted water, cook orzo for 10 minutes or until al dente.

2. Meanwhile, in a skillet, heat oil over high heat for 30 seconds; add onions and cook, stirring, for 1 or 2 minutes or until slightly charred. Remove from heat and set aside.

3. When the orzo is cooked, drain well and transfer to casserole. Add sautéed onions to orzo and stir to combine. Add tomatoes and tomato sauce; mix thoroughly. Add cooked beans; fold until evenly distributed.

4. Cover the orzo mixture and bake, covered, for 30 minutes. Remove from oven and mix in tomato juice. Top with Parmesan shavings and return to the oven, uncovered, for another 10 to 12 minutes or until the cheese is melted. Serve on pasta plates, making sure each portion is topped with some of the melted cheese. Drizzle a few drops of extra virgin olive oil on each portion and garnish with chopped parsley. Serve immediately, with Romano as an optional accompaniment.

Baked beans with molasses and ham over small shell pasta

Serves 4

If you've got 2 or 3 hours to spare, you can make a tasty pot of old-fashioned baked beans. Or you can take a few shortcuts — as I've done here — and still end up with a great result! Store-bought cooked ham gives this dish a smoky-salty flavor that's delicious with the beans-and-molasses combination. Who needs all the fatty bacon that comes with traditional baked beans?

PREHEAT OVEN TO 400° F (200° C)
SMALL BAKING DISH

1 cup	dried navy or pea beans, rinsed and drained *or* 2 3/4 cups [675 mL] canned cooked beans, drained	250 mL
1 cup	chopped onions	250 mL
1 1/2 tsp	minced garlic	7 mL
4 oz	cooked ham, chopped	125 g
1 1/4 cups	beef or chicken stock	300 mL
1/2 cup	tomato pasta sauce	125 mL
1/4 cup	ketchup	50 mL
1/3 cup	molasses	75 mL
1/4 cup	packed brown sugar	50 mL
8 oz	small shell pasta	250 g

1. If using cooked beans, proceed to step 2. Otherwise, in a saucepan over medium-high heat, cover uncooked beans with cold water; bring to a boil. Reduce heat; simmer for 5 minutes. Remove from heat; let stand, covered, for 1 hour. Drain beans. Return to saucepan; cover with cold water. Bring to a boil; reduce heat to medium. Cook, covered, for 1 hour or until tender; drain.

2. In a nonstick saucepan sprayed with vegetable spray, cook onions and garlic over medium-high heat for 3 minutes or until softened. Add ham, stock, pasta sauce, ketchup, molasses and brown sugar; bring to a boil. Pour ham mixture and beans into baking dish; bake, covered, in preheated oven for 20 minutes.

3. Meanwhile, in a large pot of boiling water, cook pasta for 8 to 10 minutes or until tender but firm; drain. In a serving bowl combine pasta and bean mixture; toss well. Serve immediately.

Three-cheese creamy pasta bean bake

Serves 6

Tip

Fettuccine, spaghetti or small shell pasta can replace linguine.

Try other bean combinations such as chickpeas, navy beans or black beans.

Replace Italian seasoning with dried basil.

Make Ahead

Prepare all elements of recipe, except for pasta, up to 2 days in advance.

Assemble early in the day, then bake.

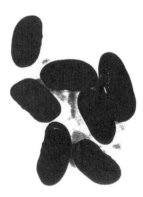

PREHEAT OVEN TO 350° F (180° C)

8-CUP (2 L) CASSEROLE DISH SPRAYED WITH VEGETABLE SPRAY

1 cup	shredded part-skim mozzarella cheese (about 4 oz [125 g])	250 mL
1 cup	5% ricotta cheese	250 mL
3/4 cup	light sour cream	175 mL
1/4 cup	2% milk	50 mL
2 tbsp	grated Parmesan cheese	25 mL
8 oz	linguine, broken into thirds	250 g
2 tsp	vegetable oil	10 mL
1 1/2 tsp	minced garlic	7 mL
1 cup	chopped onions	250 mL
1/2 cup	chopped green bell peppers	125 mL
2 cups	prepared tomato pasta sauce	500 mL
3/4 cup	canned red kidney beans, rinsed and drained	175 mL
3/4 cup	canned white kidney beans, rinsed and drained	175 mL
2 tsp	Italian seasoning	10 mL
Topping		
1/3 cup	dry seasoned bread crumbs	75 mL
4 tsp	grated Parmesan cheese	20 mL
2 tsp	olive oil	10 mL

1. In a small bowl, stir together mozzarella, ricotta, sour cream, milk and Parmesan; set aside.

2. In a pot of boiling water, cook linguine for 8 to 10 minutes or until tender but firm. Rinse under cold running water, drain and stir into cheese mixture.

3. In a nonstick saucepan sprayed with vegetable spray, heat oil over medium-high heat. Add garlic, onions and green peppers; cook 3 minutes or until softened. Stir in tomato sauce, red kidney beans, white kidney beans and Italian seasoning; reduce heat to low and cook for 5 minutes.

4. Meanwhile, make the topping: In a small bowl, combine bread crumbs, Parmesan cheese and olive oil; set aside.

5. Spoon one-half of pasta-cheese mixture into prepared casserole; top with half of bean mixture. Repeat layers. Sprinkle with bread crumb topping. Bake for 25 minutes or until golden and hot.

Cracked wheat and lima bean wrap

Makes 10 wraps

Tip
This makes enough filling for 10 large wraps so if you don't have a large crowd to feed, make half the recipe or freeze leftover filling.

Variations
Substitute: Sour cream for yogurt; 1 1/2 cups (375 mL) cooked lentils or chickpeas for lima beans.

Omit: Olives and lettuce, if desired.

2 tbsp	olive oil	25 mL
1 cup	chopped onions	250 mL
2	cloves garlic, minced	2
1 cup	chopped celery	250 mL
2 tbsp	finely chopped preserved ginger	25 mL
1 tsp	ground cumin	5 mL
1 tbsp	ground turmeric	15 mL
1 cup	cracked wheat	250 mL
3 tbsp	fresh lemon juice	45 mL
1	can (28 oz [796 mL]) stewed tomatoes	1
1	can (19 oz [540 mL]) lima beans, drained and coarsely chopped	1
	Salt and black pepper	
2/3 cup	plain yogurt	150 mL
10	large flour tortillas	10
1 cup	sliced black olives	250 mL
2 cups	shredded lettuce	500 mL

1. In a large skillet, heat oil over medium-low heat. Cook onions and garlic for 10 minutes or until soft. Add celery; cook, stirring often, for 3 minutes. Add ginger, cumin and turmeric; cook for 2 minutes.

2. Stir in cracked wheat, lemon juice and tomatoes, breaking up tomatoes with back of a spoon. Simmer over low heat, covered, for 20 minutes or until liquid is absorbed and wheat is tender.

3. Remove from heat; stir in lima beans. Season to taste with salt and pepper. Allow to cool to room temperature or store in refrigerator for up to 3 days.

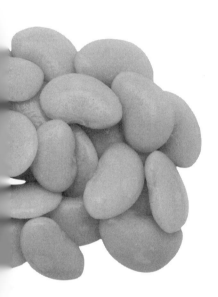

4. Spread 1 tbsp (15 mL) yogurt on each tortilla. Spoon about 1/2 cup (125 mL) filling down center of each wrap. Top with 1 rounded tbsp (15 mL) olives and 3 tbsp (45 mL) lettuce. Fold bottom up and both sides in, leaving top open. Fold in half. Serve slightly warm.

Savory chicken fagioli over rigatoni

Serves 6

Ever wonder what goes into chili powder? Well, there's ground chilies (no surprise there), but also a number of other spices common to Southwestern-style cooking. These often include cumin, ginger, cayenne, oregano and dried mustard. But since there is no one formula for chili powder, the actual ingredients vary with different brands. I find that those from the smallest producers are the most flavorful.

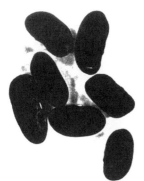

1/2 cup	chopped carrots	125 mL
1/2 cup	chopped onions	125 mL
1/3 cup	chopped celery	75 mL
1 1/2 tsp	minced garlic	7 mL
1	can (19 oz [540 mL]) red kidney beans, rinsed and drained, half the amount mashed	1
1	can (19 oz [540 ml]) tomatoes, with juice	1
2/3 cup	chicken stock	150 mL
2 tsp	packed brown sugar	10 mL
1 1/2 tsp	dried basil	7 mL
1 tsp	chili powder	5 mL
1 tsp	dried oregano	5 mL
1	bay leaf	1
12 oz	skinless boneless chicken breast, diced	375 g
12 oz	rigatoni	375 g
1/4 cup	grated low-fat Parmesan cheese	50 mL
1/4 cup	chopped fresh parsley	50 mL

1. In a large nonstick saucepan sprayed with vegetable spray, cook carrots, onions, celery and garlic over medium-high heat for 4 minutes or until softened. Add mashed beans, whole beans, tomatoes, chicken stock, brown sugar, basil, chili powder, oregano and bay leaf. Bring to a boil; reduce heat to medium-low. Cook for 20 minutes or until vegetables are tender, stirring occasionally to break up tomatoes. Add chicken; cook for 3 minutes or until cooked through.

2. Meanwhile, in a large pot of boiling water, cook rigatoni for 10 to 12 minutes or until tender but firm; drain.

3. In a serving bowl, combine pasta and sauce; toss well. Sprinkle with Parmesan cheese and parsley. Serve immediately.

Meatless

Serves 4

Barbecued tempeh with basil, hyssop and ginger

Tip

Commercial barbecue sauces are high in sugar, salt and preservatives. The sauce in this recipe offers the medicinal qualities of fresh, wholesome ingredients. Make double batches when tomatoes are at their peak and freeze in small amounts.

Hyssop is a perennial herb, native to central and southern Europe, but grown in North America. It is useful in treating coughs, bronchitis, fevers and sore throats. You can purchase fresh or dried sprigs in alternative/health stores — or you can grow your own!

Variations

Substitute: Organic barbecue sauce (available at alternative/health stores) for barbecue sauce made in recipe; Maple syrup or molasses for ginger syrup; More or less cayenne pepper, to taste.

PREHEAT OVEN TO 400° F (200° C)
SHALLOW BAKING PAN, LIGHTLY GREASED

Barbecue Sauce

6	tomatoes	6
1	onion, quartered	1
1	head garlic	1
3 tbsp	olive oil	45 mL
1/3 cup	ginger syrup	75 mL
	Salt and black pepper	
1/2 cup	stock	125 mL
1/4 cup	apple cider vinegar	50 mL
2 tbsp	fresh lemon juice	25 mL
1 tbsp	soya sauce	15 mL
1	can (5 1/2 oz [156 mL]) tomato paste	1
1 tsp	mustard powder	5 mL
6	fresh thyme leaves	6
1	sprig rosemary	1
1	sprig sage	1
1 tsp	cayenne pepper (or to taste)	5 mL

Tempeh

1 cup	Barbecue Sauce (from recipe above)	250 mL
3	sprigs basil, shredded	3
3	sprigs hyssop, shredded	3
2 tbsp	chopped candied ginger	25 mL
4	squares frozen tempeh	4
	Fresh basil or hyssop sprigs for garnish	

1. Using a sharp knife, core tomatoes, cut in half, gently squeeze out seeds and liquid. Arrange halves in prepared baking pan, cut-side down. Add onion wedges to pan.

2. Rub loose skin from outside of garlic; cut 1/4 inch (1 cm) off top and place, cut-side up, on baking pan with tomatoes and onion. Drizzle with oil.

3. Bake in preheated oven for 45 to 60 minutes or until garlic is very soft and onions are browned (tomatoes will be full of liquid). Remove from oven; allow to cool slightly. Remove tomato skins.

4. Squeeze roasted garlic cloves into a food processor or blender. Add roasted onions, tomatoes with their liquid and ginger syrup; process until smooth. Season to taste with salt and pepper, if desired.

5. Transfer purée to a saucepan; add stock, vinegar, lemon juice, soya sauce, tomato paste, mustard, thyme leaves, rosemary, sage and cayenne. Simmer for 15 minutes. Use sauce immediately or allow to cool. Keep in refrigerator no longer than 1 week, or freeze in 1-cup (250 mL) quantities.

6. In a small bowl, combine 1 cup (250 mL) barbecue sauce, basil, hyssop and ginger.

7. In a shallow baking dish, arrange tempeh squares in a single layer. Pour barbecue sauce over; marinate for at least 2 hours at room temperature or in refrigerator overnight.

8. Preheat barbecue to medium-high. Lift squares out of marinade and grill, basting occasionally, for 3 minutes per side. Heat marinade and drizzle over tempeh to serve. Garnish with sprigs of fresh basil or hyssop.

Chickpea-herb burgers

Makes 6 burgers

Tip
Whether grilled on the barbecue or baked in the oven, these burgers are great with all the trimmings.

Variations
Substitute: Rolled oats for spelt flakes.

PREHEAT OVEN TO 375° F (190° C) OR GRILL TO HIGH
PARCHMENT-LINED BAKING SHEET OR GREASED GRILL

1 tbsp	vegetable oil	15 mL
1	can (19 oz [540 mL]) chickpeas, drained	1
1/2 cup	grated onions	125 mL
2	cloves garlic, minced	2
3 cups	shredded carrots	750 mL
1/2 cup	spelt flakes	125 mL
1/4 cup	unblanched almonds	50 mL
1/4 cup	sunflower seeds	50 mL
2 tbsp	flax seeds	25 mL
2 tbsp	chopped parsley	25 mL
2 tbsp	basil leaves	25 mL
1 tbsp	fresh thyme leaves	15 mL
1	egg	1
	Salt and black pepper	

1. In a food processor or blender, purée oil, chickpeas, onions, garlic and carrots until well combined.

2. Add spelt flakes, almonds, sunflower seeds, flax seeds, parsley, basil, thyme and egg. Process until finely chopped and holding together. Season to taste with salt and pepper if desired.

3. Form mixture into 6 patties, Arrange patties on prepared baking sheet or grill. Bake in preheated oven or grill for 3 minutes per side, being careful to turn burgers gently.

Quick curried lentils

Serves 4 to 6

With a vegetarian in the family, I count on this Indian-inspired dish with its bold seasonings as a reliable main-course dish. A bowlful makes a quick and easy supper.

Tip

For a meat-lover's version of this dish, add chopped left-over roast lamb, roast beef or baked ham for the last 10 minutes of cooking.

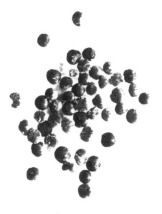

1 tbsp	vegetable oil	15 mL
1	medium onion, chopped	1
3	cloves garlic, finely chopped	3
1 tbsp	minced ginger root (or 1 tsp [5 mL] ground ginger)	15 mL
2 tsp	ground cumin	10 mL
1 tsp	ground coriander	5 mL
1 cup	green lentils, washed and sorted	250 mL
1	can (19 oz [540 mL]) tomatoes, chopped	1
1 1/2 cups	vegetable stock *or* chicken stock	375 mL
1/3 cup	chopped fresh coriander or parsley	75 mL
	Salt and black pepper	

1. In a large saucepan, heat oil over medium heat. Add onion, garlic, ginger, cumin and coriander; cook, stirring, for 3 minutes or until softened.

2. Add lentils, tomatoes and stock. Bring to a boil; reduce heat, cover and simmer for 35 minutes or until lentils are tender. Stir in coriander; season to taste with salt and pepper.

Falafel burgers with creamy sesame sauce

Serves 4

Tip
Replace coriander with dill or parsley.

Peanut butter can replace tahini.

Make Ahead
Prepare burgers early in the day and refrigerate until ready to cook. Prepare sauce up to a day ahead.

2 cups	drained canned chickpeas	500 mL
1/4 cup	chopped green onions	50 mL
1/4 cup	chopped fresh coriander	50 mL
1/4 cup	finely chopped carrots	50 mL
1/4 cup	bread crumbs	50 mL
3 tbsp	lemon juice	45 mL
3 tbsp	water	45 mL
2 tbsp	tahini (puréed sesame seeds)	25 mL
2 tsp	minced garlic	10 mL
1/4 tsp	ground black pepper	1 mL
Sauce		
1/4 cup	light sour cream	50 mL
2 tbsp	tahini	25 mL
2 tbsp	chopped fresh coriander	25 mL
2 tbsp	water	25 mL
2 tsp	lemon juice	10 mL
1/2 tsp	minced garlic	2 mL
2 tsp	vegetable oil	10 mL

1. Put chickpeas, green onions, coriander, carrots, bread crumbs, lemon juice, water, tahini, garlic and black pepper in food processor; pulse on and off until finely chopped. With wet hands, form each 1/4 cup (50 mL) into a patty.

2. In a small bowl, whisk together sour cream, tahini, coriander, water, lemon juice and garlic.

3. In a nonstick skillet sprayed with vegetable spray, heat 1 tsp (5 mL) of oil over medium heat. Add 4 patties and cook for 3 1/2 minutes or until golden; turn and cook for 3 1/2 minutes longer or until golden and hot inside. Remove from pan. Heat remaining 1 tsp (5 mL) oil and cook remaining patties. Serve with sesame sauce.

Hummus and sautéed vegetable wraps

Serves 4

Tip

Flavored tortillas — such as pesto, sun-dried tomato, herb or whole wheat — are now appearing in many supermarkets. The different colors make these wraps an attractive dish for entertaining.

Try substituting other herbs — such as coriander, basil or parsley — for the dill.

If tahini is unavailable, use peanut butter.

Make Ahead

Prepare hummus up to 3 days in advance.

Sauté vegetables early in day and reheat before serving.

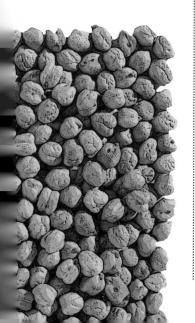

1 cup	canned chickpeas, rinsed and drained	250 mL
1/4 cup	tahini	50 mL
1/4 cup	water	50 mL
2 tbsp	freshly squeezed lemon juice	25 mL
4 tsp	olive oil	20 mL
1 tbsp	chopped fresh parsley	15 mL
3/4 tsp	minced garlic	4 mL
2 tsp	vegetable oil	10 mL
1 cup	diced onions	250 mL
1 1/4 cups	diced red bell peppers	300 mL
1 1/4 cups	chopped snow peas	300 mL
1/4 cup	chopped fresh dill (or 2 tsp [10 mL] dried)	50 mL
4	10-inch (25 cm) flour tortillas, preferably different flavors, if available	4

1. Make the hummus: In a food processor, combine chickpeas, tahini, water, lemon juice, oil, parsley and garlic; process until creamy and smooth. Transfer to a bowl and set aside

2. In a large nonstick saucepan, heat oil over medium-high heat. Add onions and sauté 4 minutes or until soft and browned. Add red peppers and sauté 4 minutes or until soft. Add snow peas and sauté for 2 minutes or until tender-crisp. Stir in dill and remove from heat.

3. Divide hummus equally among tortillas, spreading to within 1/2 inch (1 cm) of edge. Divide vegetable mixture between tortillas. Form each tortilla into a packet by folding bottom edge over filling, then sides, then top, to enclose filling completely.

Judi's enchiladas

Serves 4

This vegetarian Tex-Mex palate-rouser is yet another memento of my long and fondly remembered collaboration with Judi Roe, the superchef of southwestern Quebec. We often used to serve this dish to film crews if it was summer and we could feed them outdoors on picnic tables, instantly igniting a southern ambience.

Corn tortillas are best in this recipe.

Vegans or calorie-conscious types can easily omit both cheese and sour cream, for a leaner but just as delicious meal.

PREHEAT OVEN TO 350° F (180° C)
RECTANGULAR BAKING DISH (ABOUT 9 BY 13 INCHES [25 BY 45 CM]),
LIGHTLY GREASED WITH VEGETABLE OIL

3 tbsp	vegetable oil	45 mL
1 tbsp	chili powder	15 mL
Pinch	salt	Pinch
1	onion, finely diced	1
2	cloves garlic, minced	2
1 cup	double-strength vegetable stock	250 mL
1 cup	tomato juice	250 mL
1 tsp	cornstarch	5 mL
1 tbsp	water	15 mL
1	medium tomato, skinned, seeded and finely chopped	1
8 oz	potatoes, boiled and cubed (about 2)	250 g
2 cups	cooked romano beans	500 mL
1 1/2 cups	grated cheese (Monterey Jack or medium Cheddar cheese)	375 mL
12	small tortillas (about 6 inches [15 cm]), preferably corn	12
1/2 cup	sour cream (optional)	125 mL
	Few sprigs fresh coriander, chopped	

1. Make the sauce: In a saucepan heat vegetable oil over high heat for 30 seconds. Add chili powder and salt and stir for 30 seconds (the oil will turn vibrantly red). Add onion and stir-fry for 2 minutes or until softened. Add garlic and stir-fry for 1 minute. Add vegetable stock and tomato juice and bring to boil, stirring. Reduce heat to medium-low and cook, stirring occasionally, for 4 to 5 minutes. Dissolve cornstarch in water; add to sauce, stirring briskly, and cook until the sauce has the consistency of thin syrup. Stir in the tomatoes and remove from heat.

2. Make the filling: In a bowl combine potatoes, beans and grated cheese, folding gently so as to mix thoroughly without mashing potato or beans. Set aside.

3. Assemble the enchiladas: Grasp a tortilla firmly by one edge, dunk in the sauce to coat it, then place it in baking dish. Spoon 1/3 cup (75 mL) of the filling down the center of the tortilla middle and roll it up like a cigar. Repeat filling procedure with remaining tortillas.

4. Pour remaining sauce evenly over the enchiladas and bake for about 15 minutes or until heated through. Divide enchiladas between 4 dinner plates (3 each) and top with 1 to 2 tbsp (15 to 25 mL) of the sour cream, if using. Garnish with coriander and serve with rice and salad.

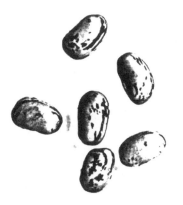

Bean burgers with dill sauce

Serves 8 or 9

Tip
Serve in a pita or tortilla with lettuce, tomatoes and onions.

Another simple topping can be made with 3 parts 2% yogurt and 1 part Dijon mustard.

Substitute black beans with another bean of your choice.

Make Ahead
Prepare mixture and sauce up to 1 day in advance. Reheat gently.

PREHEAT OVEN TO 425° F (220° C)
BAKING SHEET SPRAYED WITH VEGETABLE SPRAY

Burgers

2 cups	canned black beans, rinsed and drained	500 mL
1/2 cup	dry seasoned bread crumbs	125 mL
1/3 cup	chopped fresh dill	75 mL
1/3 cup	chopped red onions	75 mL
1/4 cup	finely chopped carrots	50 mL
2 tbsp	cornmeal	25 mL
1	egg	1
1 1/2 tsp	minced garlic	7 mL
1/4 tsp	salt	1 mL

Sauce

3 tbsp	light sour cream	45 mL
2 tbsp	light mayonnaise	25 mL
2 tsp	freshly squeezed lemon juice	10 mL
1/4 to 1/2 tsp	minced garlic	1 to 2 mL
1 tbsp	chopped fresh dill (or 1/2 tsp [2 mL] dried)	15 mL

1. In a food processor, combine black beans, bread crumbs, dill, onions, carrots, cornmeal, egg, garlic and salt. Pulse on and off until well combined. With wet hands, scoop up 1/4 cup (50 mL) of mixture and form into a patty. Put on prepared baking sheet. Repeat procedure for remaining patties. Bake in preheated oven for 15 minutes, turning at the halfway point.

2. Meanwhile, make the sauce: In a small bowl, stir together sour cream, mayonnaise, lemon juice, garlic and dill. Serve burgers hot with sauce on side.

Spicy rice, bean and lentil casserole

Serves 4 to 6

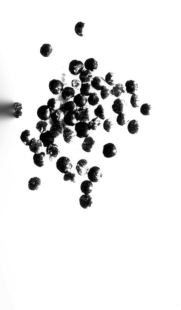

2 tsp	vegetable oil	10 mL
2 tsp	minced garlic	10 mL
1 cup	chopped onions	250 mL
3/4 cup	chopped green bell peppers	175 mL
3 3/4 cups	vegetable stock	950 mL
3/4 cup	brown rice	175 mL
1/2 cup	green lentils	125 mL
1 tsp	dried basil	5 mL
1 tsp	chili powder	5 mL
1	can (19 oz [540 mL]) red kidney beans, rinsed and drained	1
1 cup	canned or frozen corn kernels, drained	250 mL
1 cup	medium salsa	250 mL

1. In a nonstick saucepan, heat oil over medium-high heat. Add garlic, onions and green peppers; cook for 3 minutes. Stir in stock, brown rice, lentils, basil and chili powder; bring to a boil. Reduce heat to medium-low and cook, covered and stirring occasionally, for 30 to 40 minutes or until rice and lentils are tender and liquid is absorbed.

2. Stir in beans, corn and salsa; cover and cook for 5 minutes or until heated through.

Chickpea tofu burgers with coriander mayonnaise

Serves 4 to 5

PREHEAT OVEN TO 425° F (220° C)
BAKING SHEET SPRAYED WITH VEGETABLE SPRAY

1 cup	canned chickpeas, rinsed and drained	250 mL
8 oz	firm tofu	250 g
1/3 cup	dry bread crumbs	75 mL
2 tbsp	tahini	25 mL
1 1/2 tbsp	freshly squeezed lemon juice	20 mL
1 tsp	minced garlic	5 mL
1	egg	1
1/4 tsp	freshly ground black pepper	1 mL
1/4 tsp	salt	1 mL
1/3 cup	chopped fresh coriander	75 mL
1/4 cup	chopped green onions	50 mL
1/4 cup	chopped red bell peppers	50 mL
Sauce		
1/4 cup	2% plain yogurt	50 mL
1/4 cup	light sour cream	50 mL
1/4 cup	chopped fresh coriander	50 mL
1 tbsp	light mayonnaise	15 mL
1/2 tsp	minced garlic	2 mL

1. In a food processor, combine chickpeas, tofu, bread crumbs, tahini, lemon juice, garlic, egg, pepper and salt; process until smooth. Add coriander, green onions and red peppers; pulse on and off until well-mixed. With wet hands, scoop up 1/4 cup (50 mL) of mixture and form into a patty. Put on prepared baking sheet. Repeat procedure for remaining patties. Bake in preheated oven for 20 minutes, turning burgers at halfway point.

2. Meanwhile, make the sauce: In a small bowl, stir together yogurt, sour cream, coriander, mayonnaise and garlic; set aside. Serve burgers hot with sauce on side.

Serves 6 to 8

Vegetarian shepherd's pie with peppered potato topping

Tip

This shepherd's pie rivals the beef version — creamy, thick and rich tasting. Beans provide the meat-like texture.

For a different twist, try sweet potatoes.

Try other cheeses such as mozzarella or Swiss.

Make Ahead

Prepare up to 1 day in advance. Reheat gently.

Freeze for up to 3 weeks.

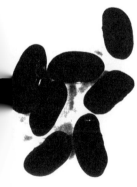

PREHEAT OVEN TO 350° F (180° C)

13- BY 9-INCH (3 L) BAKING DISH

2 tsp	vegetable oil	10 mL
2 tsp	minced garlic	10 mL
1 cup	chopped onions	250 mL
3/4 cup	finely chopped carrots	175 mL
1 1/2 cups	prepared tomato pasta sauce	375 mL
1 cup	canned red kidney beans, rinsed and drained	250 mL
1 cup	canned chickpeas, rinsed and drained	250 mL
1/2 cup	vegetable stock *or* water	125 mL
1 1/2 tsp	dried basil	7 mL
2	bay leaves	2
4 cups	diced potatoes	1 L
1/2 cup	2% milk	125 mL
1/3 cup	light sour cream	75 mL
1/4 tsp	freshly ground black pepper	1 mL
3/4 cup	shredded Cheddar cheese	175 mL
3 tbsp	grated Parmesan cheese	45 mL

1. In a saucepan heat oil over medium-high heat. Add garlic, onions and carrots; cook 4 minutes or until onions are softened. Stir in tomato sauce, kidney beans, chickpeas, stock, basil and bay leaves. Reduce heat to medium-low and cook, covered, for 15 minutes or until vegetables are tender. Remove bay leaves. Transfer sauce to a food processor; pulse on and off just until chunky. Spread over bottom of baking dish.

2. Place potatoes in a saucepan and add cold water to cover; bring to a boil. Reduce heat and simmer for 10 to 12 minutes or until tender. Drain; mash with milk, sour cream and pepper. Spoon on top of sauce in baking dish. Sprinkle with Cheddar and Parmesan cheese. Bake, uncovered, for 20 minutes or until hot.

Zucchini, mushroom and bean loaf with tomato sauce

Serves 6 to 8

PREHEAT OVEN TO 350° F (180° C)
9- BY 5-INCH (2 L) LOAF PAN SPRAYED WITH VEGETABLE SPRAY

1 tsp	vegetable oil	5 mL
2 tsp	minced garlic	10 mL
1 cup	chopped onions	250 mL
1/2 cup	finely chopped carrots	125 mL
2 cups	chopped zucchini	500 mL
1 cup	chopped mushrooms	250 mL
1 1/2 cups	canned chickpeas, rinsed and drained	375 mL
1 1/2 cups	canned white kidney beans, rinsed and drained	375 mL
1/3 cup	dry seasoned bread crumbs	75 mL
3 tbsp	chili sauce	45 mL
2 tbsp	grated Parmesan cheese	25 mL
2	eggs	2
1 tsp	dried basil	5 mL
3/4 cup	prepared tomato pasta sauce	175 mL

1. In a nonstick frying pan, heat oil over medium-high heat. Add garlic, onions and carrots; cook 4 minutes. Stir in zucchini and mushrooms; cook for 8 minutes or until softened.

2. In a food processor, combine zucchini mixture, chickpeas, white kidney beans, seasoned bread crumbs, chili sauce, Parmesan cheese, eggs and basil. Pulse on and off until finely chopped and well combined. Press into prepared loaf pan.

3. Bake, uncovered, for 40 minutes or until tester inserted in center comes out clean. Heat tomato sauce and serve with sliced loaf.

Tip

This is my favorite vegetarian loaf, which tastes a lot like chicken.

The combination of puréed beans provides a meaty texture.

Replace bottled chili sauce with barbecue sauce or ketchup.

This loaf is a good source of fiber.

Make Ahead

Prepare up to 1 day in advance and serve cold or reheated.

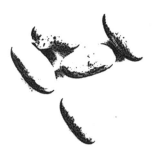

Black bean, corn and leek frittata

Serves 4 to 6

Tip
Here's a great variation on the traditional omelet — but with less fat and cholesterol.

Replace beans and vegetables with other varieties of your choice.

Coriander can be replaced with dill, parsley and basil.

Make Ahead
Combine entire mixture early in the day. Cook just before serving.

1 1/2 tsp	vegetable oil	7 mL
2 tsp	minced garlic	10 mL
3/4 cup	chopped leeks	175 mL
1/2 cup	chopped red bell peppers	125 mL
1/2 cup	canned or frozen corn kernels, drained	125 mL
1/2 cup	canned black beans, rinsed and drained	125 mL
1/3 cup	chopped fresh coriander	75 mL
2	eggs	2
3	egg whites	3
1/3 cup	2% milk	75 mL
1/4 tsp	salt	1 mL
1/4 tsp	freshly ground black pepper	1 mL
2 tbsp	grated Parmesan cheese	25 mL

1. In a nonstick saucepan sprayed with vegetable spray, heat oil over medium-high heat. Add garlic, leeks and red peppers; cook 4 minutes or until softened. Remove from heat; stir in corn, black beans and coriander.

2. In a bowl whisk together whole eggs, egg whites, milk, salt and pepper. Stir in cooled vegetable mixture.

3. Spray a 12-inch (30 cm) nonstick frying pan with vegetable spray. Heat over medium-low heat. Pour in frittata mixture. Cook for 5 minutes, gently lifting sides of frittata to let uncooked egg mixture flow under frittata. Sprinkle with Parmesan cheese. Cover and cook another 3 minutes or until frittata is set. Slip frittata onto a serving platter. Cut into wedges and serve immediately.

Fragrant Thai vegetarian curry

Serves 4 to 5

Coconut milk-based curries are a major part of Thai cuisine. Curry pastes are elaborate mixtures of fresh and dry herbs and seasonings that are time-consuming to make. We are fortunate that commercially prepared basic curry pastes are available here. Most grocers will carry at least green and red curry pastes. This vegetarian curry uses green curry paste as its base. The commercially prepared paste will most likely have some shrimp paste in it and therefore is not strictly vegetarian; for vegetarians, I give an alternative homemade paste recipe (see Variation). I also include a basic Thai vegetable stock.

When preparing curries, it is always preferable to add stock to the coconut milk, lending complexity and depth to the sauce. Other types of vegetable stock can be used or, for non-vegetarians, chicken stock would be good here.

My restaurant version of this dish features 3 kinds of eggplant: Asian purple eggplant, small green round eggplants and green wild pea eggplants. Vary the vegetables to taste and according to season, and try to vary the colors. Thai curries are generally quite soupy, with lots of sauce to eat with fragrant Thai white rice.

10 oz	Chinese bean curd or firm tofu	300 g
2 tsp	vegetable oil	10 mL
4 tsp	Thai green curry paste	20 mL
1	stalk lemon grass, cut into short lengths	1
1 tsp	palm sugar or light brown sugar or white sugar	5 mL
1/2 tsp	salt	2 mL
1	can (14 oz [400 mL]) coconut milk	1
1/2 cup	vegetable stock or chicken stock	125 mL
3	kaffir lime leaves, deveined and halved or 2 strips lime peel	3
1 cup	oyster mushrooms or other type	250 mL
1 cup	cubed calabasa or other orange-fleshed squash (such as butternut or acorn)	250 mL
10	stalks asparagus, peeled and cut into thirds	10
1	Asian eggplant, halved and cut lengthwise into wide slices	1
1	zucchini, halved and cut lengthwise into wide slices	1
12	Thai basil leaves or other basil leaves	12
1/2 tsp	lime juice	2 mL
	Coriander sprigs for garnish	

1. Rinse bean curd; drain and weigh down with a plate for 30 minutes to extract extra water. Cut into cubes. (If preferred, the bean curd can be lightly browned in oil before cutting into cubes.)

2. In a saucepan, heat oil over medium heat; cook curry paste and lemon grass until fragrant. Stir in sugar and salt. Gradually stir in coconut milk, stock and lime leaves; bring to a boil. Reduce heat and simmer for 5 minutes. Stir in mushrooms, squash, asparagus, eggplant, zucchini and bean curd. Return to a boil; reduce heat to medium and cook, covered, for 10 minutes or until vegetables are tender. Stir in basil. Remove from heat; stir in lime juice. Serve with white rice and garnished with coriander.

FAGIOLI ALLA TOSCANA (WHITE BEANS WITH TOMATO) (PAGE 175) ➢

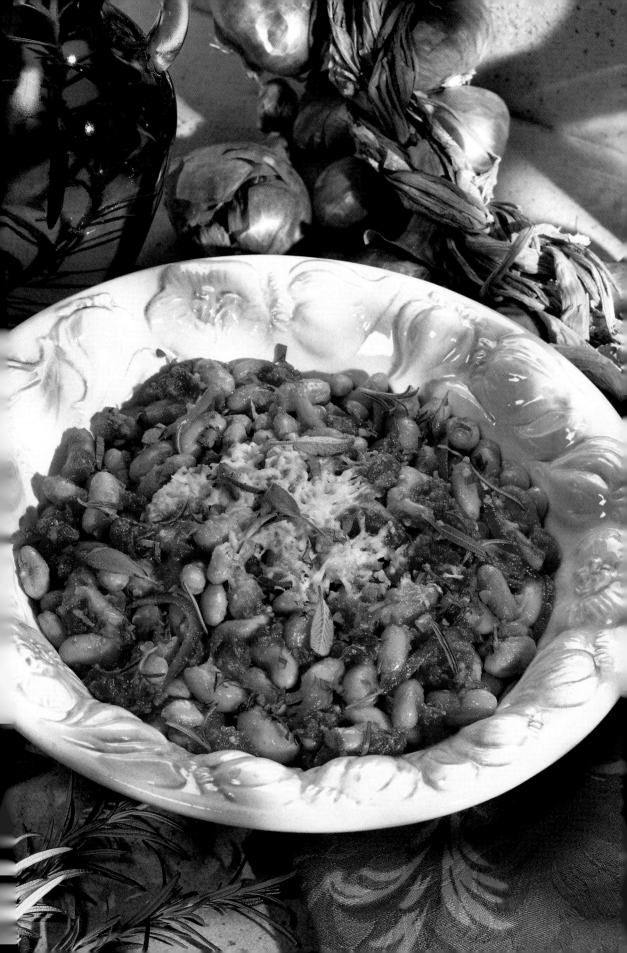

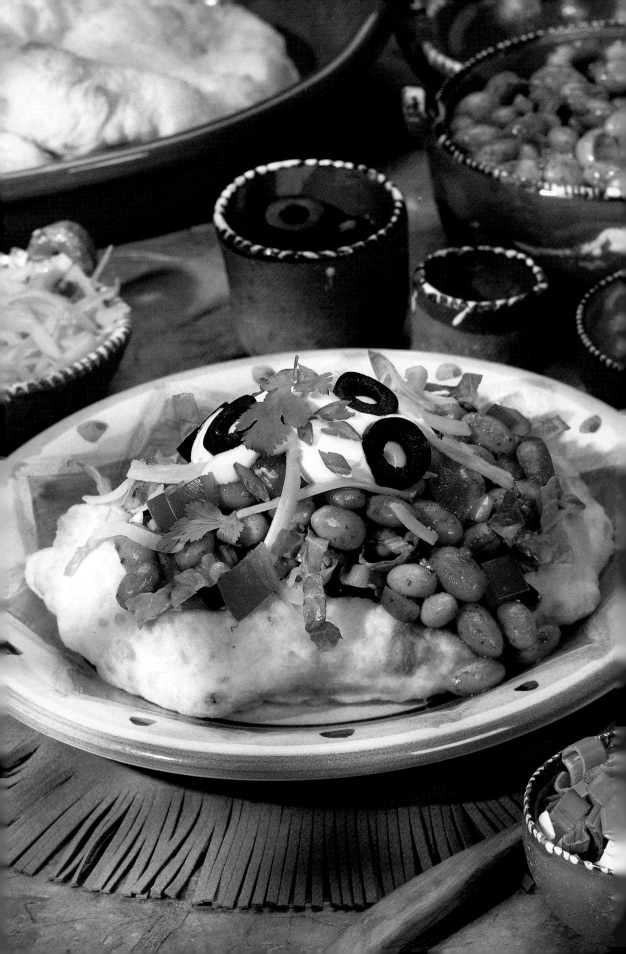

Thai vegetable stock

Variation

To make your own curry paste (enough for 3 curries): In a food processor or blender, combine 1 tbsp (15 mL) oil, 2 tbsp (25 mL) finely chopped lemon grass, 4 cloves garlic, 5 small shallots, 1 1/2 tsp (7 mL) chopped galangal or ginger root, 1 stalk coriander including roots, 1/2 tsp (2 mL) grated kaffir lime or lime rind, 10 green bird-eye chilies, 1 very finely chopped or pounded fresh bay leaf or 1/4 tsp (1 mL) ground dried bay leaf, 1 tsp (5 mL) each ground toasted coriander, cumin and fennel seeds, 1/4 tsp (1 mL) ground black pepper, 1/8 tsp (0.5 mL) ground cloves and 3/4 tsp (4 mL) salt; process to form a fine paste. Store extra paste, well covered, in refrigerator for 2 weeks or frozen for up to 6 months.

1 tbsp	vegetable oil	15 mL
1	onion, sliced	1
1	1-inch (2.5 cm) piece ginger root, smashed with the of a knife	1
1	stalk coriander, including roots	1
1	stalk lemon grass, bruised and cut into short lengths	1
15	black peppercorns	15
2	cloves	2
1	tomato, quartered	1
1	Asian eggplant or half regular eggplant, sliced and soaked in cold water for 30 minutes	1
2 cups	coarsely shredded Napa cabbage and/or lettuce	500 mL
1 cup	mushrooms stems or pieces	250 mL
1 tsp	salt	5 mL

1. In a large saucepan, heat oil over medium heat. Add onion, ginger, coriander, lemon grass, peppercorns and cloves; cook until fragrant and onion is softened. Stir in 8 cups (2 L) water, tomato, drained eggplant, cabbage, mushrooms and salt. Bring to a boil; reduce heat to simmer and cook for 1 1/2 hours. Strain, discarding solids. Stock will keep for 1 week in refrigerator or freeze in small portions for later use.

◄ INDIAN FRYBREAD TOSTADAS (PAGE 178)

Serves 4 to 6 as a shared course

This is a peculiarly Thai cooking method, where crisp, separately fried ingredients are cooked together with curry paste, sugar and fish sauce to make a dry curry. The dish incorporates a bit of oil, but the end result should not be greasy.

In Thailand, fish is sometimes added to this type of preparation, as are fried lotus seeds and/or salted duck egg yolks. I have come up with my own combination of vegetables that I think complement each other well and are readily available at regular grocery stores. Cut each vegetable into a different shape to keep them distinct; all should be cut fairly thin but not less than 1/8 inch (5 mm).

Variation
For stronger basil flavor, fry half the basil leaves for garnish and add the remaining leaves to the curry with the red chili rings.

Thai dry vegetable curry

1	small onion, thinly sliced	1
1/2 tsp	salt	2 mL
2 cups	vegetable oil	500 mL
2	carrots, cut crosswise into thirds and thinly sliced lengthwise	2
1	kohlrabi, cut in half and sliced into half-rounds	1
1	large baking or frying potato, cut into round slices or taro root	1
1 1/2 cups	canned bamboo shoots, rinsed, drained and sliced	375 mL
1 cup	Chinese bean curd or firm tofu, cut into rectangles or square slices	250 mL
2/3 cup	loosely packed Thai or holy basil	150 mL
2 tbsp	Thai red curry paste	25 mL
2 tbsp	granulated sugar	25 mL
4 tsp	fish sauce	20 mL
1 or 2	red finger chilies, sliced into rings	1 or 2

1. In a bowl combine onion and salt; set aside for 30 minutes. Drain, discarding liquid. Pat onion slices dry with paper towel.

2. In a wok or deep saucepan, heat oil to 350° F (180° C). Cook onion until golden and crisp; remove with slotted spoon and drain on paper towel. Cook separately the carrot, kohlrabi, potato, bamboo shoots and tofu in the hot oil until golden and crisp; drain on paper towel. Remove all but 1/3 cup (75 mL) of the oil. Fry basil leaves until crispy but not browned; remove immediately from hot oil and drain on a paper towel.

3. Add curry paste to oil; cook until fragrant. Stir in sugar and fish sauce; mix well. Add vegetables (except onion and basil); cook, stirring constantly, until curry paste adheres to all the vegetables. Add chili rings; mix. Serve garnished with fried onions and basil.

Side dishes

Leek-potato-lentil pie

Serves 4

The subtly flavored filling of this pie highlights the sweet, earthy tastes of its main ingredients. It is made with no dairy products at all and can be enjoyed vegan-style.

Be sure to wash leek thoroughly, splitting down the middle and paying special care to the grit that hides where the green and white parts meet.

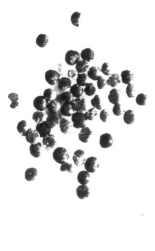

PREHEAT OVEN TO 400° F (200° C)
4 RAMEKINS, 1 1/2-CUP (375 ML) CAPACITY, MEASURING
1 TO 2 INCHES (5 CM) DEEP AND 5 INCHES (12.5 CM) WIDE

1/4 cup	olive oil	50 mL
1/4 tsp	salt	1 mL
1/4 tsp	black pepper	1 mL
8 oz	boiled potatoes (about 2), cubed	250 g
2	leeks, green and white parts alike, finely chopped	2
1/2 cup	tomato sauce	125 mL
1 1/2 cups	tomato juice	375 mL
2 cups	cooked lentils	500 mL
1 cup	thinly shredded spinach, packed	250 mL
1/4 cup	finely chopped fresh parsley	50 mL
4	sheets OLIVE OIL CRUST (see recipe, facing page)	4
1	egg	1
1 tbsp	milk	15 mL

1. In a large, deep frying pan, heat olive oil over high heat. Add salt and pepper and stir. Add potatoes and leeks. Actively stir-fry for 5 minutes or until leeks have cooked down to 1/4 of their original volume.

2. Add tomato sauce and tomato juice; stir to bring back to a boil. Reduce heat to medium. Add lentils and cook, stirring, for 5 minutes or until everything is piping hot and well mixed. Add chopped spinach, turn a few times and transfer mixture to a bowl. Add chopped parsley and mix in. Let mixture cool down for about 20 minutes, uncovered and unrefrigerated.

3. Put one quarter of the mixture (about 1 1/4 cups [300 mL]) into each ramekin. Cover the filling with a sheet of crust, pinching the excess pastry to the outside edges of rims. Whisk together the egg and milk and brush over the crusts. Bake for 20 to 22 minutes or until golden brown and crusty.

Olive oil crust

Makes 4 small crusts

This is an all-purpose crust for savory pies and serves as a serious competitor to store-bought phyllo. It is easy to work with: trimmings can be re-rolled with no loss, and it lives happily in the fridge for up to 5 days. It can also be frozen, but must be fully defrosted, and the oil that will have seeped out must be worked back into the dough.

1 3/4 cups	all-purpose flour	425 mL
1 1/2 tsp	salt	7 mL
1 1/2 tsp	baking powder	7 mL
1/2 cup	olive oil	125 mL
1/2 cup	milk	125 mL
1	whole egg, beaten	1
	Additional flour (as needed)	

1. In a bowl sift together flour, salt and baking powder. In a separate bowl, whisk together olive oil, milk and beaten egg. Add the liquid ingredients all at once to the dry ingredients. Using fingers or an electric mixer with dough hook, blend the liquids into the flour. (If you use a mixer, scrape down the sides of the bowl several times.) This shouldn't take long; the dough will have absorbed the liquids and have the texture of an earlobe. If dough does not have the correct texture, work in another 2 tbsp (25 mL) flour.

2. Transfer the dough to a storage bowl, cover and refrigerate for at least 1/2 hour. When ready to use, knead any oil that may have seeped out back into the dough.

3. To roll crusts for making pies, divide the dough into 4 equal pieces. On a floured work surface, take one piece of dough and flatten it into a round with your hand. Turn it over and flour the other side. Using a floured rolling pin, roll dough into a round sheet about 8 or 9 inches (19 or 22 cm) in diameter and about 1/8 inch (2 mm) thick. It will shrink a little on its own, but can be stretched by hand later. Transfer onto a piece of waxed paper. Repeat procedure for 3 remaining pieces of dough and stack them, separated by waxed paper, to ensure that they peel off easily when ready to use. The stack can then be covered and refrigerated.

Serves 6 to 8

Butter beans and grilled red pepper

This recipe combines the soft sweetness of beans with the pungency of grilled red peppers and chunks of tomato.

Butter beans are known as dried lima beans in the American South.

Just about any large bean, or assortment of beans, may be substituted for butter beans in this recipe.

3	red bell peppers, grilled, seeded and cut into strips	3
1	large white onion, peeled, halved and thinly sliced	1
1	clove garlic, minced	1
3	cans (each 19 oz [540 mL]) butter beans, rinsed and drained	3
2 cups	canned Italian plum tomatoes, drained, seeded and chopped	500 mL
1/2 cup	chopped flat leaf parsley	125 mL
3 tbsp	extra virgin olive oil	45 mL
1/4 cup	fresh lemon juice	50 mL
1 tsp	finely grated lemon zest	5 mL
	Salt and freshly ground black pepper, to taste	

1. In a large bowl, combine red peppers, onion, garlic, beans, tomatoes and parsley. Toss to combine well.

2. In a small bowl, whisk together olive oil, lemon juice, lemon zest, salt and pepper. Pour over bean mixture; stir to combine. Cover bowl with plastic wrap; let stand for 30 minutes at room temperature. Serve.

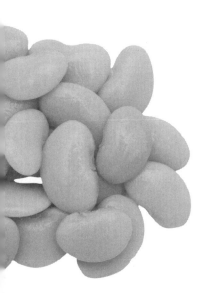

Frijoles borrachos Mexicanos

Serves 8

Borrachos means "drunken" in Spanish and, in this recipe, refers to the fact that both tequila and beer lend their special qualities to the humble pinto bean. Very good with warmed tortillas or as a side dish with Mexican-style grilled fish.

Pinto is Spanish for "painted" — an apt description for these beans, which feature streaks of reddish-brown. Along with pink beans, these are the beans most commonly used in the making of refried beans.

Look for cans of chipotle chili peppers (smoked jalapeños) in the international section of large supermarkets or in Mexican or Latin American markets.

1 lb	dried pinto beans	500 g
1 1/2 cups	Mexican beer	375 mL
5 cups	water	1.25 L
2	chipotle chili peppers, seeded and finely chopped	2
4	cloves garlic, minced	4
1 tsp	cumin seeds, toasted	5 mL
2 tbsp	vegetable oil	25 mL
1	onion, chopped	1
2	cloves garlic, minced	2
4	tomatoes (fresh or canned), chopped	4
2	fresh jalapeños, seeded and chopped	2
	Salt and freshly ground black pepper, to taste	
1/2 cup	tequila	125 mL
1 cup	chopped fresh coriander	250 mL

1. In a colander rinse pinto beans, discarding any stones. Transfer beans to a large pot. Add beer, water, chipotles, garlic and cumin seeds; bring to a boil. Reduce heat and simmer gently, covered, for 1 to 1 1/2 hours or until tender.

2. Meanwhile, heat oil in a skillet over medium heat. Add onion and garlic; cook for 5 minutes or until softened. Add tomatoes, jalapeños, salt and pepper. Simmer, stirring occasionally, for 5 minutes or until thickened. Remove from heat.

3. When beans are done, stir in tomato mixture and tequila; simmer for 5 to 10 minutes. Remove from heat and stir in coriander. Serve immediately.

Spinach dal

Serves 6

This flavorful, soothing and very nutritious Indian lentil (*dal*) recipe shows the flip-side of chef Kamala McCarthy's spicy cooking. She serves it over rice with a vegetable curry for a balanced meal. Kamala prefers to use *chana dal*, which requires 1 hour of soaking and 1 1/2 hours of cooking. Instead, I've chosen *masoor dal*, the tiny red lentil that needs next to no soaking and cooks quickly. Admittedly, I lose the nuttier texture of the *chana*, but I gain the creamy, rich consistency of the smaller lentil, as well as its vibrant color.

Ghee (clarified butter) can be purchased at East Indian specialty shops or made at home by heating butter over low heat (without boiling it) and skimming off whey as it rises to the surface.

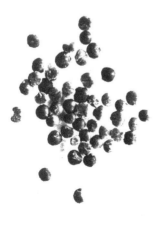

3 1/2 cups	*masoor dal* (red lentils), rinsed and drained	875 mL
8 cups	water	2 L
1 tbsp	turmeric	15 mL
1 tsp	whole cloves	5 mL
3	bay leaves	3
2 tbsp	*ghee* (clarified butter)	25 mL
2	onions, finely chopped	2
2 tbsp	minced ginger root	25 mL
5	cloves garlic, minced	5
6 cups	chopped fresh spinach, packed down	1.5 L
1 tbsp	salt	15 mL
1/4 cup	*ghee* (clarified butter)	50 mL
1 tsp	black mustard seeds	5 mL
1 tsp	whole cumin seeds	5 mL
4 tsp	garam masala	20 mL
2 tbsp	chopped fresh coriander	25 mL
	Steamed rice	

1. Put *dal* and water into a large pot and bring to a boil. Remove from heat. Add turmeric, cloves and bay leaves and stir. Let sit for 10 to 15 minutes or until *dal* has swollen and soaked up much of the water.

2. Place the lentil pot over high heat and cook, stirring occasionally, for 5 to 7 minutes or until bubbling. Reduce heat to medium and cook, stirring occasionally, for another 15 to 20 minutes or until the *dal* is tender. (If the *dal* dries out, add 1 to 2 cups [250 to 500 mL] boiling water.)

3. Meanwhile, in a frying pan heat the *ghee* over high heat for 30 seconds. Add onions and stir-fry for 2 minutes. Add ginger and garlic and stir-fry for another 2 minutes. Remove from heat and add to the *dal*. Continue cooking the *dal* with its new additions for 5 minutes, stirring occasionally. Add spinach strips and salt; cook, stirring well, for 10 minutes.

4. Meanwhile, in a small saucepan heat *ghee* over medium heat for 1 minute. Add the mustard and cumin seeds. Stir-fry for 2 to 3 minutes or until the seeds begin to pop. Add this mixture to the simmering *dal*. The hot fat will hit the wet lentils with a distinct sizzle (this is called a "chaunk"). Stir, and add 3 tsp (45 mL) of the garam masala. Stir again, reduce heat to medium-low and cook for 5 minutes, stirring occasionally.

5. Remove from heat and let rest uncovered for 15 minutes. Transfer to a serving bowl, sprinkle with the remaining garam masala and the coriander. Serve accompanied by steamed rice.

Yahni
Greek beans with onions

Serves 6

The affinity of beans to onions is no culinary secret, but this heirloom recipe stretches the notion to its limits. A mixture of approximately equal amounts of onion to beans, it is further onion-enhanced with a garnish of raw onion at the end. It results in a sweet, satisfyingly flavored bean dish that can be used on the side of any Mediterranean main course.

If using canned kidney beans, a 19-oz (540 mL) can of beans, rinsed and drained, will yield the 2 cups (500 mL) required for this recipe.

2	medium tomatoes	2
1/4 cup	olive oil	50 mL
1/4 tsp	salt	1 mL
1/4 tsp	black pepper	1 mL
2 cups	thinly sliced onions	500 mL
1	stick celery, finely diced	1
4	cloves garlic, thinly sliced	4
1 cup	water	250 mL
1/4 cup	chopped fresh parsley, packed down	50 mL
1 tbsp	red wine vinegar	15 mL
1 tsp	sugar	5 mL
2 cups	cooked white kidney beans	500 mL
	Extra virgin olive oil, to taste	
1/4 cup	finely diced red onions	50 mL

1. Blanch tomatoes in boiling water for 30 seconds. Over a bowl, peel, core and deseed them. Chop tomatoes into chunks and set aside. Strain any accumulated tomato juices from bowl; add the juices to the tomatoes.

2. In a large frying pan, heat oil over high heat for 30 seconds. Add salt and pepper and stir. Add onions and celery and stir-fry for 5 minutes or until wilted. Add garlic and stir-fry for 1 minute or until garlic is well coated with oil and everything is shiny.

3. Add tomato and its juices. Stir-fry for 2 minutes, mixing well. Add water, parsley, vinegar and sugar; bring back to a boil. Reduce heat to medium-low and cook for 5 to 6 minutes. Stir occasionally, mashing the tomato until it has broken down and the sauce is pink.

4. Fold beans into the sauce. Cook, stirring occasionally (and gently), for 5 to 6 minutes or until most of the liquid has been absorbed and everything is well integrated.

5. Transfer to a serving dish. Drizzle with virgin olive oil and top with red onions. Let rest covered and unrefrigerated for 1 to 2 hours to develop flavor. Serve at room temperature.

Lentils-rice-spinach

Serves 4 to 6

This is a variation of spanako-rizo (spinach-rice), a rustic winter staple of the eastern Mediterranean, where spinach is one of the leafy vegetables that keep growing in the cold months. The lentils are my own addition, but they are in keeping with the traditions of this kind of cuisine. They also bolster this dish into main-course status.

The lentils-rice-spinach can be served immediately, or it can wait for up to 2 hours, covered and unrefrigerated.

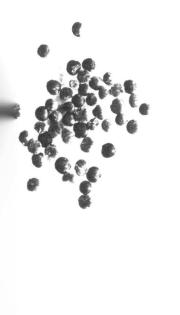

1/4 cup	olive oil	50 mL
1/4 tsp	salt	1 mL
1/4 tsp	black pepper	1 mL
2 cups	diced onions	500 mL
1	medium tomato, cubed	1
4 cups	chopped fresh spinach leaves, packed down	1 L
1 1/2 cups	cooked rice (from 1/2 cup [125 mL] raw rice)	375 mL
2 cups	cooked green lentils	500 mL
1	lemon, cut into wedges	1

1. In a pot or large skillet, heat oil over high heat for 30 seconds. Add salt and pepper and stir for 30 seconds. Add onions and stir-fry for 2 minutes or until softened. Add cubed tomato and stir-fry for 1 minute.

2. Add all the spinach at once; cook, turning over several times, for 1 minute or until the spinach has been reduced to one third of its volume.

3. Reduce heat to medium-low and add rice and lentils. Stir-cook for 3 to 4 minutes or until well mixed and everything is piping hot. Remove from heat, cover and let rest for 5 to 6 minutes as it develops flavor. Serve with lemon wedges on the side.

Pea tops with pancetta and tofu

Serves 4

Pea tops are the shoots of snow pea plants. They're now available almost year round in Asian markets. They are tasty in salads and have a subtle, nutty flavor when cooked. However, they are quite perishable and won't last much longer than a couple of days in your refrigerator.

1	3-inch (7.5 cm) square medium tofu	1
2 tbsp	vegetable oil, divided	25 mL
	Salt and pepper to taste	
1 tsp	sesame oil	5 mL
2	slices pancetta or prosciutto, finely chopped	2
2 tsp	minced garlic	10 mL
8 oz	pea tops or arugula	250 g
2 tbsp	chicken stock or vegetable stock	25 mL

1. Slice tofu into pieces 1/2 inch (1 cm) thick by 1 1/2 inches (3.5 cm) square.

2. In a nonstick skillet, heat 1 tbsp (15 mL) oil over medium-high heat for 30 seconds. Add tofu and season lightly with salt, pepper and sesame oil; fry 1 minute per side or until golden. Remove from skillet; arrange on a platter and keep warm.

3. Add remaining oil to skillet and heat for 30 seconds. Add pancetta and garlic; fry briefly for 20 to 30 seconds or until fragrant. Add pea tops and stock; stir-fry until pea tops are just wilted. Arrange evenly over tofu and serve.

Serves 4

Soy-braised tofu, cabbage and ginger with cellophane noodles

Braising is a key component of Chinese cooking — it adds rich flavor to otherwise bland ingredients such as tofu. Baking also firms the tofu and allows the flavorings to penetrate.

For added flavor, roast the cabbage along with the tofu.

Bean thread noodles are very slippery and best eaten with chopsticks.

PREHEAT OVEN TO 375° F (190° C)
GREASED BAKING SHEET

4 oz	bean thread noodles *or* 8 oz (250 g) dried angel hair pasta	125 g
4 oz	medium-firm tofu, cut into 1/2-inch (1 cm) cubes	125 g
1 tbsp	vegetable oil, plus oil for coating noodles	15 mL
2 tbsp	soya sauce	25 mL
2 tbsp	minced ginger root	25 mL
1 tbsp	minced garlic	15 mL
4 cups	vegetable stock *or* apple juice	1 L
2 cups	shredded green cabbage	500 mL
1 tbsp	chopped cilantro	15 mL
2 tbsp	tomato ketchup	25 mL
1 tbsp	horseradish	15 mL
1 tbsp	cornstarch dissolved in 2 tbsp (25 mL) water	15 mL
	Salt and pepper to taste	

1. In a heatproof bowl or pot, cover noodles with boiling water and soak for 3 minutes. Drain. (If using pasta, prepare according to package directions and coat with a little oil.) Set aside.

2. In a large bowl, combine tofu, oil, soya sauce, ginger and garlic. Place on a baking sheet and roast for 15 minutes or until firm and browned. Remove from oven and allow to cool slightly.

3. Meanwhile, in a saucepan over medium-high heat, combine stock, cabbage, tofu mixture, cilantro, ketchup and horseradish. Bring to a boil. Reduce heat and simmer for 5 minutes. Add dissolved cornstarch and cook until mixture begins to thicken. Add noodles and stir until heated through. Season with salt and pepper; serve immediately.

Tomatoes stuffed with corn, black beans and pine nuts

Serves 4

4	medium tomatoes	4
1/2 cup	canned corn kernels, drained	125 mL
1/2 cup	canned black beans, rinsed and drained	125 mL
1/4 cup	chopped fresh coriander	50 mL
1/4 cup	chopped green onions	50 mL
1/4 cup	chopped red bell peppers	50 mL
2 tbsp	light mayonnaise	25 mL
2 tbsp	toasted pine nuts	25 mL
1 tbsp	grated Parmesan cheese	15 mL
2 tsp	freshly squeezed lemon juice	10 mL
1 tsp	Dijon mustard	5 mL

1. Slice tops off tomatoes and reserve. Scoop out and discard seeds and core.

2. In a small bowl, mix together corn, black beans, coriander, green onions, red peppers, mayonnaise, pine nuts, Parmesan, lemon juice and Dijon.

3. Divide mixture evenly between tomato shells, about 1/3 cup (75 mL) per tomato. Cover with reserved tomato tops and serve.

Tip

These stuffed tomatoes are visually stunning. Serve as an appetizer or a side vegetable dish.

If black beans are unavailable, use chickpeas or white navy beans.

The filling is great as a salad by itself.

Make Ahead

Prepare filling up to 1 day in advance. Stuff tomatoes a few hours before serving.

Fagioli alla toscana
White beans with tomato

Serves 4 to 6

Turn leftovers into a fabulous soup the day after enjoying these flavorful Tuscan-style baked beans scented with fresh rosemary and enriched with Pecorino Romano.

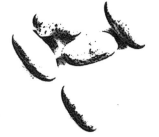

PREHEAT OVEN TO 375° F (190° C)
8-CUP (2 L) CASSEROLE WITH LID

1/4 cup	olive oil	50 mL
1/4 cup	chopped flat-leaf parsley	50 mL
8	fresh sage leaves	8
2	branches rosemary	2
4	cloves garlic, finely chopped	4
1 cup	canned Italian plum tomatoes, chopped, with juices	250 mL
	Salt and freshly ground black pepper	
2 cups	dried cannellini (white kidney beans) or navy beans, soaked overnight in water to cover	500 mL
1 cup	grated Pecorino Romano	250 mL

1. In a large skillet, heat olive oil over medium-low heat. Add parsley, sage, rosemary and garlic; cook, stirring occasionally, for 6 minutes or until the garlic is softened and the herbs are fragrant. Stir in tomatoes with juice and a pinch each of salt and pepper; cook for 3 minutes or until slightly thickened.

2. In casserole dish, stir together tomato mixture, drained beans and half of the Pecorino Romano. Add enough cold water to cover beans; stir well. Cover casserole and bake for 2 1/2 hours or until beans are tender, testing for doneness every 30 minutes. (Cooking time will depend on freshness of the beans.)

3. Remove and discard rosemary branches, which should be bare. Sprinkle remaining cheese over the surface. Cook, uncovered, for 10 minutes longer or until cheese is golden. Serve from casserole.

Serves 4 to 6

Lenticchie in umido
Lentils cooked with wine and tomato

The best lentils for this dish are the little dark green ones called *cavellucchi* in Italy and *puy* in France. They remain firm during cooking — unlike the conventional orange or pale green lentils, which become a little too mushy.

2 tbsp	olive oil	25 mL
2	cloves garlic, finely chopped	2
1	onion, finely chopped	1
1	carrot, finely chopped	1
1 1/2 cups	lentils (see note at left), soaked in cold water overnight	375 mL
1 cup	dry red wine	250 mL
1 cup	passata (puréed, sieved tomatoes) *or* canned ground plum tomatoes	250 mL
1 cup	chicken stock *or* vegetable stock	250 mL
1/2 tsp	salt	2 mL
1/4 tsp	freshly ground black pepper	1 mL
1 lb	spinach	500 g

1. In a large skillet, heat olive oil over medium-high heat. Add garlic, onion and carrot; cook, stirring occasionally, for 7 minutes or until vegetables are softened. Stir in drained lentils; cook 2 minutes longer.

2. Pour in wine. Bring to a boil; boil for 2 minutes. Reduce heat to medium-low. Stir in passata, stock, salt and pepper. Cover and cook, stirring occasionally, for 20 minutes or until lentils are tender. Meanwhile, prepare spinach.

3. Trim and wash spinach. Put the spinach in a large saucepan with just the water that clings to the leaves after washing. Cook, covered, over high heat until steam begins to escape from beneath lid. Remove lid, toss spinach and cook 1 minute or until tender. Remove from heat. Drain, pressing spinach against sides of colander to squeeze out as much water as possible. Chop spinach roughly. Set aside.

4. When lentils are tender, stir in spinach. Adjust seasoning as necessary and serve.

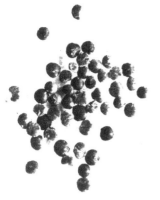

Serves 4 to 6

Here's a pleasant combination of flavors that, once prepared, can be enjoyed as is or tossed with cooked pasta. This preparation works very well with large lima beans if fava beans are not available.

Fresh young fava (or broad beans) do not need their individual husks or skins peeled; if they look as though they do, they are too old. However, there are those who maintain that the inner skin of each bean should be removed — it's a matter of personal taste.

Fave con pancetta
Fava beans with bacon

1 tbsp	extra virgin olive oil	15 mL
4 oz	pancetta, diced	125 g
1	onion, thinly sliced	1
1	stalk celery, chopped	1
1 lb	shelled young fresh fava beans (about 3 lbs [1.5 kg] unshelled fava beans)	500 g
1 cup	beef stock	250 mL
	Salt and freshly ground black pepper	
2 tbsp	chopped flat-leaf parsley	25 mL

1. In a large skillet, heat olive oil over medium heat. Add pancetta, onion and celery; cook, stirring often, for 8 minutes or until vegetables are softened.

2. Stir in fava beans and beef stock. Bring to a boil, reduce heat to medium-low and cook, uncovered and stirring occasionally, for 25 minutes or until beans are tender. Season to taste with salt and pepper. Stir in parsley and serve immediately.

Indian frybread tostadas

Serves 8

Frybread or bannock is always found at Native pow-wows and at rodeos like the Calgary Stampede, where you can have it hot and sprinkled with sugar. Natives throughout the West, from prairie Blackfoot tribes to the Navajo in Arizona, rely on frybread as a daily staple. This dish is a kind of tostada, with beans (or you can use ground beef), lettuce, toma-toes, cheese and guacamole piled high on a piece of warm frybread.

Frybread

3 cups	all-purpose flour (or half white and half whole wheat)	750 mL
1 tsp	baking powder	5 mL
1 tsp	salt	5 mL
Pinch	granulated sugar (optional)	Pinch
1 cup	warm milk	250 mL
1 tsp	canola oil	5 mL
	Canola oil for frying	

Toppings

1 tbsp	canola oil	15 mL
2	cloves garlic, minced	2
1	onion, chopped	1
1	green bell pepper, chopped	1
2	cans (each 19 oz [540 mL]) pinto beans, rinsed and drained	2
1/4 cup	tomato sauce *or* ketchup *or* bottled barbecue sauce	50 mL
1 tbsp	chili powder	15 mL
1 tsp	ground cumin	5 mL
1 cup	shredded lettuce	250 mL
1 cup	chopped tomato	250 mL
1 cup	shredded sharp Cheddar cheese	250 mL
1/2 cup	low-fat sour cream	125 mL
1/4 cup	sliced black olives	50 mL
1/4 cup	chopped cilantro	50 mL
1/4 cup	chopped green onions	50 mL

1. **Frybread:** In a large bowl, stir together flour, baking powder, salt and, if using, sugar. Stir in the warm milk and oil, mixing with a wooden spoon. Stir in just enough warm water to make a soft but not sticky dough, up to 1/2 cup (125 mL). Divide dough into 8 equal pieces. Shape each piece into a 6-inch (15 cm) round, stretching and flattening dough with your hands. In a heavy frying pan, heat 1/2 inch (1 cm) canola oil over medium-high heat. One at a time, fry dough rounds 1 to 2 minutes per side or until golden brown. Drain on paper towels.

2. **Topping:** In a frying pan, heat oil over medium-high heat. Add garlic, onion and green pepper; cook for 5 minutes or until tender. Stir in beans, tomato sauce, chili powder and cumin; cook, stirring, for 2 minutes or until heated through.

3. Place frybreads on individual plates. Pile some shredded lettuce on each piece of frybread, then top with some warm bean mixture, chopped tomato and Cheddar cheese. Place a dollop of sour cream on top of the tostadas, and sprinkle each with some sliced black olives, cilantro and green onions.

Spiced rice and lentil pilaf

Serves 6

Readily available spices transform a simple rice and lentil dish into something quite exotic.

Kitchen Wisdom
You can turn this pilaf into a main course by stirring in cubes of leftover cooked poultry or meat (or cooked shrimp) about 10 minutes before the rice is ready.

Make Ahead
The pilaf can be refrigerated, covered, for up to 3 days. Reheat in the microwave on High for 6 to 8 minutes or in a 350° F (180° C) oven for 20 to 30 minutes or until piping hot.

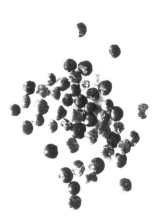

1 tbsp	canola oil *or* vegetable oil	15 mL
1	onion, chopped	1
2	cloves garlic, minced	2
1 tsp	minced ginger root	5 mL
1 tsp	turmeric	5 mL
1 tsp	ground coriander	5 mL
1 tsp	ground cumin	5 mL
1/4 tsp	salt	1 mL
1/4 tsp	black pepper	1 mL
Pinch	cayenne pepper (or more to taste)	Pinch
1 cup	green lentils, rinsed and drained	250 mL
4 cups	beef stock	1 L
1 cup	long-grain rice	250 mL
2	tomatoes, chopped	2
1/4 cup	chopped fresh mint	50 mL
1/4 cup	chopped fresh coriander or parsley	50 mL

1. In a large skillet, heat oil over medium-high heat. Add onion, garlic and ginger; cook, stirring, for 3 to 5 minutes or until onion is soft but not brown. Add turmeric, coriander, cumin, salt, pepper and cayenne; cook, stirring, for 1 minute.

2. Add lentils; stir to coat with spice mixture. Stir in stock and bring to a boil over high heat. Reduce heat to medium-low; simmer, covered, for 15 minutes.

3. Add rice. Simmer, covered, for 20 minutes or until rice and lentils are tender. Stir in tomatoes, mint and coriander. If desired, season to taste with additional salt and pepper. Transfer to a warm shallow serving dish; serve at once.

Index